Neurology

Fact

Over 200 MCQs
with explanatory answers

Ed Burton

and

Ashwin Pinto

Foreword by

Professor George Ebers

R  ess

Radcliffe Medical Press Ltd
18 Marcham Road
Abingdon
Oxon OX14 1AA
United Kingdom

www.radcliffe-oxford.com
The Radcliffe Medical Press electronic catalogue and online ordering facility.
Direct sales to anywhere in the world.

© 2004 Edward A Burton and Ashwin Pinto

Every effort has been made to ensure the accuracy of this text, and that the best information available has been used. This does not diminish the requirement to exercise clinical judgement, and neither the publishers nor the authors can accept any responsibility for its use in practice.

British Library Cataloguing in Publication Data

A catalogue record for this book is available from The British Library.

ISBN 1 85775 952 4

Typeset by Aarontype Ltd, Easton, Bristol
Printed and bound by TJ International Ltd, Padstow, Cornwall

Contents

Foreword

There is a time-honoured tradition of placing barriers in the way of physicians who wish to 'earn their spurs'. In most western countries, some form of qualifying examination is either in place or being contemplated. In this general context, the MRCP examinations are, if anything, venerable and have served a valuable purpose to generations of physicians in the UK and abroad.

Neurology as a specialty accounts relatively consistently for around 20% of patients seen in Accident and Emergency departments and in GP surgeries, but nevertheless engenders some anxiety. It is a specialty which has historically been clinical, and which seems to be perceived by students and junior doctors as an enduring legacy of clever diagnoses, flamboyant practitioners and thin therapeutics. This notion has belied an extraordinary expansion in our understanding of diseases of the nervous system which has taken place over the last decade. A useful exercise for a sceptical SHO would be to survey discharges from a neurology ward and from a cardiology ward and ask the question 'What percentage of patients were the same, better or worse as a result of their stay?'.

Regardless of the amount of neurology that the average candidate sees prior to sitting the MRCP exams, it might well dwarf the amount of formal neurology teaching that candidates receive. This book attempts to fill this gap indirectly through the process of self-assessment. Questions have been designed to maximise the amount of information that is imparted by each of the options in the '1 from 5' MCQ format, now used in MRCP and USMLE examinations. Material that lends itself to being tested in an MCQ examination is summarised in a series of tables. This should prove a useful barometer for candidates' own self-evaluation, serve to round off areas which have by chance been under-learned, and hopefully supplement and update information that has become available while candidates have been training in other specialties.

Ed Burton and Ashwin Pinto are very well qualified to write such a book, being at the end of their specialist training, having been outstanding trainees, and having had an excellent grounding in the basic and clinical sciences of the nervous system.

Professor George Ebers MD FRCPC
Professor of Clinical Neurology
University of Oxford
Oxford
September 2003

About the authors

Edward A Burton MD (Hons), DPhil, MRCP
Clinical Lecturer in Neurology
University of Oxford
Oxford

Ashwin Pinto BM, DPhil, MRCP
Specialist Registrar in Clinical Neurology
Radcliffe Infirmary
Oxford

PART 1

Symptoms and signs of neurological disease

Headache

1 Which of the following features suggests that a headache is caused by raised intracranial pressure?

a very severe pain

b association with teichopsia

c pain present on waking

d pain worse on standing

e resting tachycardia.

2 All of the following features are compatible with migraine without aura *except*:

a decreased conscious level

b photophobia

c pulsatile pain

d nausea and vomiting

e exacerbation of pain on exercise.

3   Which of the following is an effective
acute treatment for an attack of
cluster headache?

a   oral morphine

b   paracetamol

c   ibuprofen

d   pizotifen

e   oxygen.

4   All of the following are recognised
features of giant-cell arteritis (GCA)
except:

a   unilateral temporal pain

b   brainstem stroke

c   normal erythrocyte sedimentation
rate (ESR)

d   inflammatory optic neuritis

e   normal temporal artery biopsy.

1 (c)

The headache of raised intracranial pressure is not necessarily severe, but is characteristically exacerbated by lying down, and is thus often present on waking. Teichopsia (strictly a transient hemianopic defect, but often used to describe positive visual phenomena) is often part of a migrainous aura.

2 (a)

Although rarely vertebrobasilar migraine may present with loss of consciousness as part of an aura, this is very uncommon, and any alteration in conscious level should prompt a search for an alternative cause. The other features are typical of migraine headache.

3 (e)

Oral medications do not work sufficiently quickly to treat acute cluster headache attacks, which are best managed acutely with subcutaneous sumatriptan or inhaled 100% oxygen. Attacks can be prevented by oral steroids or high-dose verapamil.

4 (d)

Loss of optic nerve function is a feared complication of giant-cell arteritis, caused by anterior ischaemic optic neuropathy (not optic neuritis) secondary to vasculitis of the posterior ciliary vessels. The prognosis for recovery of vision is usually very poor. The ESR and temporal artery biopsy are not always abnormal. GCA is a recognised cause of brainstem stroke.

Quick fix: Headache diagnosis

	Migraine	Tension headache	Cluster headache	Raised intracranial pressure	Giant-cell arteritis
Site	Any; classically unilateral	Any; classically biparietal	Usually around one eye	Any	One or both temples
Character	Pulsating/throbbing	Pressure/tight	Boring/piercing	Dull	Burning/tender
Time course	Episodic; 4–72 hours in duration; may be present on waking	Episodic; 30 minutes to 7 days in duration. May be continuous or daily ('chronic tension headache'). Often worse in the evening	Episodic; 15–180 minutes in duration; frequency 0.5–8 per day; attacks occur in series lasting weeks or months ('cluster'), followed by period of months or years without attacks	Characteristically present on waking and relieved by standing; usually presents with crescendo time profile of less than 3 months	Continuous; disappears within 48 hours of starting steroid treatment
Exacerbating factors	Precipitated by alcohol or sleep disturbance. Pain worse on movement, coughing, straining or exercise	Stress	Precipitated by alcohol or sleep	Pain worse on bending, coughing or straining, after exercise and on lying down	Exacerbated by local pressure (e.g. from pillow or washing hair)
Associated symptoms	Aura (visual – teichopsia, scintillating scotomata, fortification spectra; hemisensory; other); nausea and vomiting; photophobia and phonophobia	Photophobia or phonophobia	Ipsilateral rhinorrhoea, lacrimation, sweating, nasal obstruction, eyelid swelling, ptosis	Nausea and vomiting; visual obscurations (symptoms of focal deficit or epilepsy may be present as a result of mass lesion)	Visual obscurations, skin ulceration; polymyalgia rheumatica; jaw claudication, pyrexia of unknown origin (PUO), brainstem stroke
Physical signs	None	Tenderness of upper cervical and cranial muscles	During attack: Horner's syndrome; red eye; asymmetrical flushing or sweating	Papilloedema; bradycardia; hypertension (focal signs may be present as a result of mass lesion)	Tender, pulseless, thickened temporal artery; ischaemic optic neuropathy (may have signs of brainstem stroke)

Blackouts

For each of the following clinical scenarios choose the most likely diagnosis from the list below:

a vasovagal syncope

b complex partial seizure

c hypoglycaemia

d subclavian steal syndrome

e Stokes–Adams attack

f hyperventilation

g generalised tonic–clonic convulsion

h brainstem stroke

i transient global amnesia.

5 An 80-year-old woman presents with sudden unheralded loss of consciousness that caused collapse to the ground while she was crossing the road. A witness reports that there were no limb movements, but that the patient looked very pale. She made a rapid recovery without significant confusion, tongue biting or urinary incontinence.

6 A 14-year-old schoolboy presents with a history of a flurry of blackouts which occur particularly often at school. These start with a rising sensation in his abdomen, following which he loses consciousness. His teacher reports that during each attack, which lasts for a couple of minutes, he has a 'glazed expression', makes lip-smacking movements and is unresponsive. On recovery he has a mild headache and is significantly confused and amnesic for a few minutes.

7   A 22-year-old student nurse experienced a blackout after suffering a crush injury to her hand in a car door. She experienced severe pain and remembers feeling light-headed and nauseated before losing consciousness. Her friend reported that she became pale and crumpled to the ground. There were a few asynchronous limb jerks followed by a quick return of consciousness. The patient made a rapid recovery to full consciousness and orientation.

8   A 36-year-old woman with a past history of a depressive disorder presents with episodes of attacks of altered consciousness that occur on a daily basis. Prior to each attack she feels very anxious and light-headed, and then experiences dyspnoea, 'pins and needles' in both hands together with chest discomfort. Each attack lasts for several minutes, and during the attack her husband reports that she is only partially responsive. There are no abnormal movements of the face or hands. On recovery she improves rapidly with no amnesia.

5

Blackouts are a common symptom of cardiac disease, which should be considered in their differential diagnosis, especially in the elderly. Stokes–Adams attacks are caused by sudden loss of cardiac output, most frequently due to complete heart block. A cardiovascular examination, 12-lead ECG, 24-hour ECG monitor and transthoracic echocardiogram are important investigations for identifying the cause of blackouts.

6

In contrast to primary generalised seizures, partial seizures are associated with abnormal electrographic activity arising from a focus in the cerebral cortex. A partial seizure associated with loss of awareness is called a *complex partial seizure*. The clinical characteristics vary according to the region of the brain that is affected. The case presented here is typical of seizures originating in the temporal lobe.

7

Vasovagal attacks are the commonest type of blackout in patients presenting to physicians. The circumstances surrounding the attack are important clues to the diagnosis (e.g. blackouts occurring on hot days following prolonged standing and poor fluid intake). Patients frequently report a prodrome of light-headedness, together with misting of vision, fading of hearing and nausea. A few myoclonic jerks may be seen before consciousness is recovered – this type of motor activity may be misinterpreted as indicative of an epileptic seizure. Recovery is typically very rapid, without amnesia or confusion.

8

Hyperventilation typically presents with symptoms of anxiety associated with dyspnoea, peripheral and circumoral paraesthesiae, nausea and blurred vision. There may also be partial loss of awareness. There may be a clear precipitant in some cases, and a past psychiatric history may be a clue to the diagnosis. Symptoms may be reproduced in the clinic by voluntary hyperventilation.

Quick fix: Blackout diagnosis

	Vasovagal syncope	Generalised tonic–clonic seizure	Non-epileptic attacks
Precipitant	Prolonged standing; high ambient temperature; large meal; pain	Sleep deprivation; alcohol; flashing lights	Stressful circumstances; may be induced by suggestion
Prodrome	Sweating; nausea; blurred vision; hearing fades; light-headed	May be either (i) stereotyped focal aura, or (ii) no warning	Gradual onset; non-stereotyped prodrome
Witness account	Collapse; pallor; usually motionless; occasionally clonic limb movements; unconscious for less than a minute	Tonic phase followed by synchronous clonic limb jerking; cyanosis; urinary incontinence; tongue biting; attack lasts for less than 10 minutes	No cyanosis; flailing asynchronous or bizarre limb movements; pelvic thrusting; waxing and waning attack; may be prolonged
On recovery	Rapid recovery; no post-ictal confusion; no amnesia	Prolonged recovery; drowsiness; headache; amnesia and confusion	Minimal post-ictal confusion or drowsiness

Coma

9 Which of the following is true with regard to the Glasgow Coma Scale?

a A score of less than 2 suggests a bilateral hemispheric lesion.

b Assessment of the motor response should take place on the patient's worst side.

c The scale has been universally validated as a prognostic tool for all forms of coma.

d Localisation to pain scores 5 for motor response.

e Confused speech scores 2 for verbal response.

10 Coma is characteristically caused by acute overdose with all of the following drugs *except*:

a methadone

b amitriptyline

c primidone

d paracetamol

e lorazepam.

11 For which of the following anatomical structures does damage characteristically result in coma?

a medulla oblongata

b cranio-vertebral junction

c anterior hypothalamus

d left temporal lobe

e dorsal pons.

12 Which of the following physical signs suggests that coma is caused by a focal intracerebral lesion?

a bilateral extensor plantar reflexes

b generalised hyper-reflexia

c Glasgow Coma Score of 8–11

d fever

e unilateral decerebrate posturing.

9

The Glasgow Coma Scale was developed for head injury patients, although it tends to be used to describe the conscious level of patients with many different diseases. The score is obtained by rating three different domains (speech, motor function on best side, eye opening) for spontaneous behaviour, or response to speech or pain, resulting in a maximum score of 15 (fully conscious) and a minimum score of 3 (no response to pain in any domain).

10

Acute paracetamol overdose is not dramatic clinically, although acute hepatic failure can follow after an interval, resulting in delayed hepatic coma. All of the other listed drugs characteristically cause coma in acute overdose, and clinical clues can be sought to help to identify which agent is responsible (pupils: pinpoint – opiates, dilated – tricyclics; pulse: fast and bounding – tricyclics; respiratory depression: opiates, benzodiazepines, barbiturates).

11

Level of arousal is governed by the reticular activating system (RAS) that projects from the rostro-dorsal pons diffusely throughout the hemispheres, via the upper brainstem and dorsal hypothalamus. Coma is characteristically produced by pathological processes that interfere with the functions of the RAS in the brainstem, diencephalon or both hemispheres diffusely.

12

Coma may be produced by intracranial or extracranial disease. Metabolic coma can typically produce non-localising signs, such as bilateral extensor plantars or hyper-reflexia, by diffusely affecting hemisphere and upper brainstem function. However, it is unusual for metabolic coma to be associated with localising signs, such as unilateral decerebrate posturing, which would strongly suggest a lesion of the upper brainstem or diencephalon. An exception to this general rule may be seen in hypoglycaemia, which can result in focal signs, such as hemiplegia.

Quick fix: Glasgow Coma Scale

Eye opening
Spontaneous   4
To speech   3
To pain   2
None   1

Speech
Normal   5
Confused   4
Single words   3
Incomprehensible sounds   2
None   1

Motor
Obeys commands   6
Localises to pain   5
Withdraws from pain   4
Abnormal flexion to pain   3
Extends to pain   2
None   1

Quick fix: Common causes of coma

Intracranial causes (may be associated with focal signs)

- Head injury
- Epilepsy
- Infarction (large hemisphere stroke with secondary brainstem compression, or brainstem stroke)
- Haemorrhage (intraparenchymal, pituitary, subarachnoid, subdural, extradural)
- Tumour
- Infection (abscess, empyema, encephalitis, meningitis)
- Hydrocephalus

Extracranial causes (usually not associated with lateralising signs)

- Diabetic complications (hypoglycaemia, hyperosmolar non-ketotic coma)
- Poisons and drug overdose
- Organ failure (liver, kidney, lung, adrenal, thyroid, pituitary, heart)
- Ionic disturbance (hyponatraemia, hypernatraemia, hypercalcaemia)

Vertigo, disequilibrium and dizziness

For each of the following clinical scenarios, choose the most appropriate diagnosis from the list below:

a   acute peripheral vestibular failure

b   posterior circulation stroke

c   postural hypotension

d   Ménière's disease

e   benign paroxysmal positional vertigo

f   panic attacks

g   proprioceptive loss

h   cerebellar haemangioblastoma.

13   A 74-year-old man with a past history of hypertension and ischaemic heart disease develops sudden onset of dizziness 'like being on board a ship', associated with headache, nausea and vomiting. His balance is poor, and he falls to the left. There is subjective diminution of pinprick sensation in the right arm and leg.

14   A 65-year-old man with Parkinson's disease who is on treatment with L-dopa and pergolide develops dizziness, especially first thing in the morning when getting out of bed. He describes the symptom as feeling 'woozy' or 'light-headed', and it is improved by sitting down.

15 A 24-year-old woman presents with severe dizziness which has been present since she got out of bed in the morning. She reports a sensation of the room spinning around which is present continuously but is exacerbated by head movements. She is unable to stand without losing her balance. There is associated nausea and vomiting.

16 A 48-year-old woman presents with recent development of brief episodes of dizziness. The attacks are provoked by turning to lie on her left side in bed, and by sudden movements of her head while upright. The episodes are brief, lasting less than one minute, during which time she experiences a sensation of the room spinning around.

13

Posterior circulation stroke can present with acute onset of vertigo or disequilibrium, nausea and vomiting, together with other brainstem and long-tract symptoms such as dysarthria, diplopia, facial numbness and weakness. This diagnosis should be particularly considered in the elderly with risk factors for cerebrovascular disease, such as hypertension.

14

Postural hypotension is a frequent cause of dizziness and falls in elderly patients. In this case the diagnosis is suggested by the clear history of orthostatic non-vertiginous dizziness and the presence of pathology and medications that are likely to cause or exacerbate postural hypotension.

15

Patients with acute peripheral vestibular failure present with abrupt onset of rotational vertigo associated with nausea and vomiting. Head movements exacerbate the symptoms and patients prefer to lie flat. Recovery often occurs within 5–7 days, and there is little risk of recurrence. The major differential diagnosis is of a posterior circulation infarct or a brainstem plaque from multiple sclerosis.

16

Benign paroxysmal positional vertigo is a common cause of dizziness. Patients report rotational vertigo with sudden head movements, particularly when turning in bed. The attacks are typically brief, lasting for 15–45 seconds, and may recur many times a day. The diagnosis can be confirmed by performing the Hallpike manoeuvre. This provokes acute vertigo and georotational nystagmus (fast phase towards the ground). The Epley manoeuvre can be employed to reposition the otoconial particles that are believed to be responsible for the disorder.

Quick fix: Common peripheral causes of rotational vertigo

	Benign paroxysmal positional vertigo	Acute peripheral vestibular failure	Ménière's disease
Duration	Less than a minute; many attacks per day	Several days to weeks; single prolonged episode	Up to 24 hours; attacks occur periodically
Nausea and vomiting	Rare	Common	Common
Associated signs	Hallpike's test is usually positive	Nystagmus; absent vestibulo-ocular reflex	Unilateral hearing loss

Higher mental functions

17 Which of the following statements is true with regard to disorders of speech?

a Dysarthria is often caused by ischaemic damage to the left temporal lobe.

b Dysphonia refers to inability to articulate labial and lingual consonants.

c The dysphasic patient often has difficulty in writing spontaneous prose.

d Impaired object naming is often seen in lesions of the inferior right temporal lobe.

e Expressive and receptive dysphasia rarely coexist.

18 All of the following cognitive domains may be tested to assess frontal lobe function *except*:

a phonemic fluency

b motor sequencing

c cognitive estimation

d concentration and attention

e episodic memory.

19 Which of the following suggests a diagnosis of transient global amnesia?

a   episodic memory for distant events more severely affected than that for recent events

b   amnesia, ophthalmoplegia and history of heavy alcohol consumption

c   witnessed seizure at the onset of the attack

d   moderate CSF pleocytosis

e   self-limiting episode precipitated by sudden effort.

20 Which of the following is *not* a typical clinical feature of a lesion in the left angular gyrus of a right-handed man?

a   left–right disorientation

b   acalculia

c   prosopagnosia

d   agraphia

e   finger agnosia.

17

Dysphasia describes a defect in language, which often affects spoken and written language. Inability to express and to understand language often coexist, as the brain centres responsible (the infero-lateral frontal lobe and superior temporal lobe) are close to one another, are intimately interconnected, and both are supplied by the middle cerebral artery. Dysphonia is a defect in voice production, caused by diseases that affect the larynx, and dysarthria is a defect in pronunciation of words. In both cases, the language content of speech is normal unless there is a coexisting dysphasia.

18

Episodic memory depends on the limbic circuit that encompasses the hippocampus, mamillary bodies, thalamus and cingulate gyrus in addition to parts of the temporal lobes. The other tests all tend to show impairment in patients with frontal lobe disease, although any abnormalities are not necessarily specific for frontal lobe dysfunction.

19

Transient global amnesia is characterised by a self-limiting episode lasting for a few hours in which there is retrograde amnesia for hours to weeks and complete failure to form new memory. It is often precipitated by a sudden change in ambient temperature (e.g. diving into cold water or walking out of a warm house on a winter morning) or by sexual intercourse. The cause is unknown, but it should be distinguished from other causes of acute loss of memory (see *Quick fix* opposite).

20

These are the features of Gerstmann's syndrome arising from an angular gyrus lesion in the dominant hemisphere. Prosopagnosia (inability to recognise faces despite normal visual acuity and fields) is usually the result of a lesion within the fusiform gyrus of the occipital lobe.

Quick fix: Causes of amnesia

Acute-onset, transient amnesia

- Transient global amnesia
- Epilepsy*
- Head injury
- Drugs (alcohol, benzodiazepines)
- Psychogenic

Acute-onset, persistent amnesia

- Herpes encephalitis*
- Korsakoff's syndrome*
- Subarachnoid haemorrhage (especially from anterior communicating artery aneurysm)
- Posterior cerebral artery occlusions affecting temporal lobes or thalami
- Head injury
- Anoxia
- Psychogenic

*Important treatable causes of amnesia.

Slow-onset amnesia

- Third ventricle tumours/cysts*
- Alzheimer's disease and other degenerative dementias

Visual system

21 A 24-year-old patient with intractable complex partial seizures undergoes a right temporal lobectomy for hippocampal sclerosis. What visual field defect may be present postoperatively?

a bitemporal hemianopia

b left inferior homonymous hemianopia

c left macular-sparing homonymous hemianopia

d paracentral scotoma

e left superior homonymous quadrantanopia.

22 A 42-year-old man is referred from an ophthalmology clinic with deteriorating vision. On examination he is found to have a superior bitemporal hemianopia. What is the most likely site of the lesion?

a left occipital lobe

b optic chiasm

c left optic nerve

d right parietal lobe

e bilateral parietal lobe.

23 Severe acute papilloedema is characteristically associated with:

a impaired visual acuity

b relative afferent papillary defect

c desaturation of colour vision

d enlarged blind spot

e central scotoma.

24 A left macular-sparing homonymous hemianopia is characteristically associated with:

a glaucoma

b left temporal lobe tumour

c right occipital lobe infarct

d right middle cerebral artery territory infarct

e pituitary tumour.

21

Temporal lobectomy for hippocampal sclerosis may disrupt fibres in the optic radiation as they pass through the temporal lobe (Meyer's loop), leading to contralateral homonymous superior quadrantanopia.

22

Pituitary tumours that compress the optic chiasm from below characteristically cause a bitemporal hemianopia which is initially restricted to the upper temporal quadrants.

23

Acute papilloedema is typically associated with preserved visual acuity, normal colour vision and normal visual fields except for enlargement of the blind spot. The condition should be distinguished from acute papillitis (optic neuritis with optic disc swelling), in which there is impaired visual acuity, colour desaturation, and occasionally an afferent pupillary defect.

24

Occipital lobe lesions caused by posterior cerebral artery infarcts are frequently associated with a contralateral macula-sparing homonymous hemianopia. This is believed to be due to a combination of a large macular representation in the occipital cortex and a dual blood supply from both the middle and posterior cerebral vessels.
In contrast, anterior circulation strokes caused by middle cerebral artery territory infarcts are more often associated with a contralateral macula-splitting homonymous hemianopia.

Quick fix: Causes of visual field defects

Site of pathology	Visual field defect	Common causes
Optic nerve	Central scotoma	Optic neuritis; optic nerve compression
Optic chiasm	Bitemporal hemianopia	Pituitary tumour; craniopharyngioma
Optic tract	Incongruous homonymous hemianopia	Pituitary tumour; meningioma
Optic radiation	Complete macula-splitting homonymous hemianopia	Middle cerebral artery territory stroke (TACI, PACI)
Temporal lobe	Superior quadrantic hemianopia	Space-occupying lesion; temporal lobectomy
Parietal lobe	Inferior quadrantic hemianopia	Space-occupying lesion
Occipital lobe	Homonymous hemianopia with or without macular sparing	Occipital lobe infarct or haemorrhage; space-occupying lesion

TACI, total anterior circulation infarct; PACI, partial anterior circulation infarct.

Ocular motility and pupils

25 In a lesion of the fourth cranial nerve:

a the inferior oblique muscle is the only paralysed muscle

b ocular abduction is usually impaired

c the patient characteristically experiences diplopia on tilting their head away from the side of the lesion

d partial ptosis is a frequent accompaniment

e the adducted eye fails to depress.

26 All of the following are recognised causes of a third cranial nerve palsy *except*:

a adenoma of the pituitary

b granuloma of the orbit

c angioma of the medulla oblongata

d glioblastoma of the temporal lobe

e posterior communicating artery aneurysm.

27 Which of the following features is incompatible with an isolated lesion of the third cranial nerve?

a iridoplegia

b complete ptosis

c intorsion on attempted down-gaze

d absent consensual light reflex to ipsilateral stimulus

e retention of ocular abduction.

28 Internuclear ophthalmoplegia is characterised by:

a failure of abduction and nystagmus in the adducting eye

b failure of accommodation and nystagmus in the abducting eye

c failure of adduction and iridoplegia

d failure of up-gaze and light-near dissociation of papillary response

e failure of adduction and preserved ocular vergence.

25

A fourth (trochlear) nerve palsy results in isolated paralysis of the superior oblique muscle. This muscle is responsible for depression of the adducted eye. In the neutral position of gaze, the superior oblique muscle acts with the superior rectus muscle to produce pure intorsion as part of the static vestibular–ocular reflex when the head is tilted towards the ipsilateral eye. As a result, when the superior oblique muscle is paralysed, the unopposed action of the superior rectus muscle causes the eye to elevate, resulting in vertical diplopia. This forms the basis for Bielschowsky's head-tilt test, and is the reason why patients with trochlear palsy tend to tilt their head away from the side of the lesion.

26

The third cranial nerve may be affected by pathology anywhere along its course from the midbrain to the orbit – commonly by aneurysms of the circle of Willis, uncal herniation in temporal lobe tumours and also by disruption of its blood supply in diabetes. However, it does not pass near to the medulla, so a benign medullary lesion is not a cause of third cranial nerve palsy.

27

A lesion of the third nerve causes iridoplegia, ptosis, and paralysis of all ocular movement apart from abduction (VI) and intorsion on attempted down-gaze (IV). However, the consensual light reflex (constriction of the contralateral pupil when light is shone into the ipsilateral eye) should be preserved – the afferent pathway for the reflex runs in the second cranial nerve.

28

Internuclear ophthalmoplegia is caused by a lesion in the medial longitudinal fasciculus and results in failure of adduction of the ipsilateral eye when conjugate eye movement is attempted to the opposite side. There may also be nystagmus in the abducting eye during this manoeuvre ('ataxic nystagmus'). However, adduction during vergence movement is preserved because this involves a different supranuclear pathway that does not rely on the medial longitudinal fasciculus.

Quick fix: Extra-ocular palsy

Problem	Extra-ocular movements	Pupil	Eyelid	Causes
Third nerve palsy	All movements paralysed except abduction (VI) and intorsion on down-gaze (IV)	Fixed, dilated	Complete ptosis	Aneurysm, diabetes, cavernous sinus lesion, tentorial herniation
Sixth nerve palsy	Failure of abduction	Normal	Normal	Diabetes, idiopathic, raised intracranial pressure
Fourth nerve palsy	Failure of depression in adduction; positive Bielschowsky test	Normal	Normal	Head injury
Internuclear ophthalmoplegia (INO)	Failure of adduction on attempted conjugate gaze, nystagmus in abducting eye; normal adduction on vergence	Normal	Normal	Lesion in median longitudinal fasciculus (e.g. multiple sclerosis)
Parinaud's syndrome	Failure of vergence and vertical gaze (up > down)	Fixed, dilated	Normal	Dorsal midbrain lesion (e.g. pineal tumour)
Ocular myasthenia	Any; fatiguable	Normal	May be ptosis; fatiguable	Thymoma, idiopathic

See *Quick fix* on page 65 for pupillary abnormalities

Cranial nerves V, VII and VIII

29 Which of the following muscles is supplied by the motor division of the trigeminal nerve?

a platysma

b masseter

c orbicularis oculi

d pharyngeus

e orbicularis oris.

30 Which of the following features is *not* usually seen in an isolated acute lower motor neuron facial palsy?

a impaired taste sensation on the ipsilateral side of the tongue

b hyperacusis

c weakness of platysma

d Bell's phenomenon

e ptosis.

31 A left abducens (sixth) nerve palsy in association with an acute left lower motor neuron pattern facial palsy is typically seen with a lesion in:

a left petrous temporal bone

b left pons

c left parotid gland

d right midbrain

e left internal capsule.

32 Recognised clinical features of a right acoustic neuroma include all of the following *except*:

a negative Rinne's test (i.e. bone conduction better than air conduction)

b hydrocephalus

c papilloedema

d left beating horizontal nystagmus

e impaired right corneal reflex.

29 (b)

The motor division of the trigeminal nerve supplies the muscles of mastication (medial and lateral pterygoid, masseter and temporalis) but not the muscles of facial expression (supplied by the facial nerve, VII) or the pharyngeal muscles (which are supplied by the vagus nerve, X, and cranial accessory nerve, XIc).

30 (e)

Ptosis is caused by weakness of the levator palpebrae superioris, and can be seen in lesions that affect the cranial sympathetic supply (Horner's syndrome – mild ptosis), third nerve lesions (severe ptosis) and diseases that affect the neuromuscular junction (myasthenia gravis – fatiguable ptosis) and muscle (mitochodrial myopathies). Ptosis is not a feature of facial nerve lesions.

31 (b)

A nuclear lesion of the abducens (seventh) nerve in the pons is frequently associated with an ipsilateral lower motor neuron pattern facial weakness, because the motor fibres of the facial nerve loop around the abducens nucleus before leaving the brainstem (known as the internal genu of the facial nerve; the resulting bump is macroscopically visible in the floor of the fourth ventricle – the 'facial colliculus').

32 (a)

The commonest presentation of an acoustic neuroma is progressive ipsilateral sensorineural deafness, associated with a positive Rinne's test (air conduction is greater than bone conduction). Occasionally, vertigo and tinnitus may occur. Nystagmus may be seen, typically with the fast phase away from the side of the acoustic neuroma, although other patterns occur. The corneal reflex may be lost due to compression of the adjacent trigeminal nerve in the cerebello-pontine angle. Large acoustic neuromas can also cause compression of the fourth ventricle, leading to obstructive hydrocephalus and papilloedema.

Quick fix: Distinguishing between upper and lower motor neuron facial weakness

- Upper motor neuron VII – preserved upper facial power (frontalis and orbicularis oculi); dissociation between emotional and voluntary facial expression.
- Lower motor neuron VII – complete unilateral facial weakness; loss of taste sensation on anterior two-thirds of tongue; hyperacusis.

Quick fix: Distinguishing between sensorineural and conductive deafness

Test	Normal	Sensorineural deafness	Conductive deafness
Rinne	AC > BC	AC > BC	BC > AC
Weber	Central	Contralateral to lesion	Ipsilateral to lesion

AC: air conduction (usually tested by presenting vibrating 512 Hz tuning fork to external auditory meatus, without touching patient); BC: bone conduction (usually tested by holding base of vibrating 512 Hz tuning fork firmly against patient's mastoid process).

Quick fix: Causes of cerebello-pontine-angle lesions

- Tumour (acoustic neuroma, meningioma, trigeminal or facial nerve neuromas, nasopharyngeal carcinoma).
- Vascular (basilar artery aneurysm).
- Infection (TB and syphilis).

Bulbar function

33 With regard to the gag reflex:

a the afferent pathway involves the ninth cranial nerve

b the efferent pathway involves the seventh cranial nerve

c the reflex is a useful indicator of ability to swallow

d loss of the reflex may be found in lesions of the midbrain

e in skull-base tumours, the reflex is usually lost on the contralateral side.

34 Which of the following structures does *not* enter the jugular foramen from the posterior cranial fossa?

a cranial nerve X

b the inferior petrosal sinus

c cranial nerve XI

d the sigmoid sinus

e cranial nerve XII.

35 All of the following are causes of bulbar palsy *except*:

a myasthenia gravis

b middle cerebral artery territory infarct

c Guillain–Barré syndrome

d motor neuron disease

e dermatomyositis.

36 Which of the following physical signs suggests that dysphagia is more likely to be caused by bulbar rather than pseudobulbar palsy?

a emotional lability

b brisk jaw jerk reflex

c pout reflex

d tongue fasciculation

e slow tongue movements.

33 (a)

The gag reflex is associated with elevation of the palate and constriction of the pharynx when the mucosa of the oropharynx or fauces is mechanically stimulated. The afferent pathway runs in the ninth cranial nerve and the efferent pathway involves the fifth, ninth, tenth and cranial part of the eleventh cranial nerves. The reflex is co-ordinated in the medulla, and is completely useless for predicting a patient's ability to swallow. Due to the locations of the nerves involved, the reflex may be disrupted by an ipsilateral tumour at the skull base or jugular foramen.

34 (e)

The jugular foramen contains nerves IX, X and XI along with the union of the sigmoid and inferior petrosal sinuses to form the jugular vein. Nerve XII exits the skull through the hypoglossal canal in the occipital bone.

35 (b)

Cerebrovascular disease may cause a bilateral upper motor neuron syndrome that affects the lower cranial nerves, known as pseudobulbar palsy. All of the other diseases listed can affect the motor units of the bulbar musculature, resulting in the characteristic lower motor neuron weakness of bulbar palsy. Motor neuron disease often causes a mixed picture with features of both upper and lower motor neuron involvement.

36 (d)

Tongue fasciculation is a lower motor neuron sign, suggesting bulbar palsy. The other features suggest bilateral upper motor neuron disease characteristic of pseudobulbar palsy.

Quick fix: Lower cranial nerves

	Bulbar palsy	Pseudobulbar palsy
Weakness type	Lower motor neuron	Upper motor neuron
Causes	Guillain–Barré syndrome; myasthenia gravis; dermatomyositis; motor neuron disease; brainstem stroke involving nuclei of lower cranial nerves	Bilateral strokes involving cortico-bulbar tracts in deep white matter; multiple sclerosis; motor neuron disease
Physical signs	Nasal dysarthria; dysphonia; dysphagia; wasting and fasciculation of the tongue	Dysarthria with 'strained' voice; dysphagia; small tongue with slow tongue movements; emotional lability; brisk jaw jerk; snout and rooting reflexes
Associated features	Wasting and fasciculation of the masticatory muscles (motor neuron disease); fatiguable dysarthria (myasthenia gravis); facial weakness (Guillain–Barré syndrome)	Other signs of bilateral cerebral damage (e.g. extensor plantar responses)

Quick fix: Exit foramina of cranial nerves

Nerve(s)	Foramen	Bone(s)
I	Cribriform plate	Ethmoid
II	Optic canal	Sphenoid
III, IV, Va, VI	Superior orbital fissure	Between greater and lesser wings of sphenoid
Vb	Foramen rotundum	Greater wing of sphenoid
Vc	Foramen ovale	Greater wing of sphenoid
VII	Enters temporal bone through internal auditory meatus; exits skull through stylomastoid foramen	Temporal
VIII	Internal auditory meatus	Temporal
IX, X, XI	Jugular foramen	Between temporal and occipital
XII	Hypoglossal canal	Occipital

Basal ganglia

37 Which of the following is not a recognised component of the basal ganglia?

a locus coeruleus

b substantia nigra

c subthalamic nucleus

d globus pallidus

e caudate nucleus.

38 An isolated lesion in the left subthalamic nucleus may be associated with:

a bradykinesia

b right-sided resting tremor

c left-sided weakness

d right-sided hemiballismus

e dysarthria.

39 All of the following neurotransmitters are correctly associated with projections from particular CNS nuclei *except*:

a the dorsal raphe nuclei and 5-hydroxytryptamine (5-HT)

b the substantia nigra and dopamine

c the locus coeruleus and glycine

d the putaminal projection to the internal segment of the globus pallidus and gamma-hydroxybutyric acid (GABA)

e the nucleus basalis of Meynert and acetylcholine.

40 Which of the following is *not* a characteristic symptom of basal ganglia disease?

a bradykinesia

b dystonia

c tremor

d rigidity

e muscle weakness.

37

The basal ganglia consist of five important subcortical nuclei, namely the caudate, putamen, globus pallidus, subthalamic nucleus and the substantia nigra. The locus coeruleus lies in the caudal midbrain and upper pons at the lateral margin of the periaqueductal grey matter.

38

Lesions in the subthalamic nucleus may give rise to contralateral hemiballismus. The commonest cause in adults is ischaemic stroke.

39

The forebrain projection from the locus coeruleus is predominantly noradrenergic.

40

Basal ganglia disease can present with a number of different motor symptoms, including tremor, bradykinesia, rigidity, dysarthria, chorea, dystonia and hemiballismus. Weakness is not a feature of extrapyramidal disease.

Quick fix: Causes of chorea

- Hereditary causes:
  - Huntington's disease
  - neuroacanthocytosis
  - rarely, Wilson's disease (more commonly causes tremor or dystonia)
  - other rare conditions.
- Endocrine and metabolic causes:
  - hyperthyroidism
  - pregnancy
  - hypocalcaemia
  - hypercalcaemia.

- Autoimmune causes:
  - systemic lupus erythematosus
  - antiphospholipid syndrome
  - post-infectious chorea (Sydenham's chorea).
- Drugs:
  - neuroleptics
  - levodopa
  - combined oral contraceptive.
- Vascular causes:
  - lacunar infarction.

Cerebellum

41 Which of the following statements about the afferent connections of the cerebellum is true?

a   Inputs from the inferior olivary nucleus enter through the ipsilateral middle cerebellar peduncle.

b   Inputs from the red nucleus enter through the contralateral inferior peduncle.

c   The major component of the superior peduncle is afferent and is derived from thalamic projections to the neocerebellum.

d   Neurons within the pontine nuclei give rise to fibres that decussate and enter the cerebellum via the middle peduncle.

e   The inferior peduncle contains few afferent fibres, and is composed mainly of efferent fibres projecting to the spinal cord.

42 Which of the following is a characteristic feature of a cerebellar hemisphere lesion?

a   contralateral hyper-reflexia

b   ipsilateral hypertonia

c   contralateral akinesia

d   ipsilateral dysmetria

e   contralateral paresis.

43 Which of the following is *not* a recognised cause of cerebellar ataxia?

a   chronic alcoholism

b   multiple sclerosis

c   ovarian cancer

d   hypothyroidism

e   vitamin B$_{12}$ deficiency.

44 Which of the following is *not* characteristic of alcoholic degeneration of the superior and anterior parts of the cerebellar vermis?

a   severe gaze-evoked nystagmus

b   gait ataxia that is out of proportion to heel–shin ataxia that is on the bed

c   normal arm co-ordination

d   mild dysarthria

e   wide-based stance.

41

The cerebellum connects with the rest of the CNS through white matter tracts that pass through three pairs of peduncles. The inferior peduncle mainly carries afferent tracts from the spine (dorsal spino-cerebellar tracts – ipsilateral) and the inferior olivary nucleus (crossed). The middle peduncle is dominated by afferent fibres from the pontine nuclei (crossed). The superior peduncle is the main output tract from the cerebellar deep nuclei, containing fibres that pass to the contralateral red nucleus and thalamus. The complex arrangement of crossed and uncrossed tracts means that each cerebellar hemisphere is involved in motor control of the ipsilateral side of the body.

42

Ipsilateral clinical signs of cerebellar hemisphere disease include dysmetria, intention tremor, dysdiadochokinesis, hypotonia and hyporeflexia, although the signs may be subtle even with a moderately extensive lesion. In contrast, midline lesions often produce dramatic postural instability, even in the absence of other signs.

43

All of the diseases listed can cause cerebellar ataxia, with the exception of vitamin B_{12} deficiency, which causes proprioceptive loss and sensory ataxia. Apart from the possibility of direct metastasis to the cerebellum, ovarian cancer can produce a paraneoplastic (non-metastatic, immunologically mediated) cerebellar syndrome that is associated with anti-Yo antibodies.

44

Isolated lesions of the vermis are associated with severe disequilibrium for stance, but with relative preservation of other cerebellar functions. This pattern is characteristic of alcoholic cerebellar degeneration, where severe nystagmus and dysarthria are uncommon.

Quick fix: Causes of cerebellar ataxia

Acute or subacute cerebellar ataxia

- Acute alcoholic intoxication; other drugs and toxins*
- Infarct
- Haemorrhage
- Primary or secondary neoplasm
- Multiple sclerosis
- Meningitis/encephalitis/abscess
- Wernicke's encephalopathy*

*Causes of cerebellar syndrome that is characteristically bilateral or symmetrical.

Chronic cerebellar ataxia

- Alcoholic degeneration*
- Idiopathic degeneration*
- Multiple sclerosis
- Low-grade tumour
- Paraneoplastic syndrome*
- Hypothyroidism*
- Prion disease*
- Hereditary degenerations*:
  - autosomal dominant (>15 different types, all rare, called SCA1, 2, etc.)
  - autosomal recessive (Friedreich's ataxia, Wilson's disease, ataxia telangiectasia and numerous others, all rare)

Quick fix: Eye movement disorders in cerebellar disease

- Eye movement problems in cerebellar disease are often caused by involvement of the adjacent brainstem in the pathological process.
- Lesions to the midline and paramedian cerebellar structures (flocculus, nodulus, vermis and fastigial nuclei) are particularly associated with eye movement abnormalities.
- Common abnormalities include:
  - impaired fixation
  - gaze-evoked nystagmus (fast phase towards side of lesion)
  - inaccurate saccades (hypometric – undershoot target; hypermetric – overshoot target)
  - impaired, jerky, smooth pursuit movements
  - downbeat nystagmus (flocculus and nodulus)
  - abnormalities of vestibular-ocular reflex adjustments (gain, suppression).

Spinal cord

45 Which of the following signs would *not* be expected with a right-sided intrinsic lesion in the spinal cord at T3?

a loss of pain and temperature sensation in the right leg and trunk

b weakness in the right leg

c loss of vibration sense in the right leg

d flexor plantar response on the left side

e loss of right superficial abdominal reflexes.

46 Useful clinical features for differentiating intrinsic spinal cord lesions from extrinsic compression include:

a upper motor neuron pattern weakness

b impairment of bladder function

c extensor plantar responses

d spinal pain and tenderness

e absent abdominal reflexes.

47 Which of the following findings is *not* characteristic of a cervical cord syrinx?

a extensor plantar responses

b bilateral wasting of upper limb muscles

c widespread fasciculation in lower limbs

d absent upper limb tendon reflexes

e impairment of upper limb pain and temperature sensation bilaterally.

48 A 42-year-old hypertensive man develops acute bilateral leg weakness and loss of bladder function after emergency surgery for a dissecting thoracic aortic aneurysm. The likeliest diagnosis is:

a thoracic spinal cord infarct

b acute vitamin B_{12} deficiency precipitated by nitrous oxide anaesthesia

c transverse myelitis

d extrinsic thoracic spinal cord compression

e haematomyelia.

45

A right-sided lesion in the thoracic cord will give rise to ipsilateral pyramidal weakness and dorsal column signs (joint position sense and vibration sense) and contralateral loss of pain and temperature sensation below the site of the lesion (Brown–Séquard syndrome).

46

Local pain and tenderness to palpation in the spine are suggestive of vertebral pathology, and are therefore likely to be associated with extradural compression in the context of an acute myelopathy. The other signs simply reflect damage to the spinal cord, and do not help to distinguish between compression and intrinsic pathology.

47

A cervical syrinx usually presents with symptoms suggestive of a central cord syndrome. Classically there is loss of spinothalamic function, with preservation of vibration sense and joint position sense. There may be upper motor neuron signs below the level of the syrinx, and loss of α-motor neurons at the level of the syrinx, giving rise to segmental wasting. A cervical cord syrinx may be associated with Arnold–Chiari type I malformation with descent of the cerebellar tonsils below the foramen magnum.

48

This is a classical presentation of an anterior hemi-cord syndrome due to a spinal cord infarct. Acutely, one would expect to find a flaccid paraplegia with absent lower limb reflexes (spinal shock phase), extensor plantar reflexes and loss of spinothalamic sensation, but preservation of vibration sense and proprioception.

Quick fix: Physical signs in spinal cord lesions

	Complete spinal lesion	Brown-Séquard lesion	Central cord lesion
Motor	Lower motor neuron signs in muscle groups supplied by spinal segments at site of lesion; upper motor neuron signs in muscle groups supplied by spinal segments below lesion	**Ipsilateral** lower motor neuron signs in muscle groups supplied by spinal segments at site of lesion; **ipsilateral** upper motor neuron signs in muscle groups supplied by spinal segments below lesion	Lower motor neuron signs in muscle groups supplied by spinal segments at site of lesion; upper motor neuron signs in muscle groups supplied by spinal segments below lesion
Sensory	Sensory level (may be below site of lesion)	**Contralateral** loss of spinothalamic modalities; **ipsilateral** loss of dorsal column modalities	Loss of spinothalamic modalities; relative preservation of dorsal column modalities; sensory level may be 'suspended'
Bladder involvement?	Yes	Variable	Variable

See *Quick fix* on page 165 for causes of spinal cord disease.

Upper and lower motor neuron

49 A motor unit consists of:

a a single motor neuron and its associated muscle fibre

b a group of motor neurons that innervate a muscle fascicle

c all of the motor neurons that innervate a particular muscle

d a single motor neuron and the muscle fibres that it innervates

e all of the motor neurons that innervate a single muscle fibre.

50 All of the following are characteristic features that suggest a lesion of the lower motor neuron *except*:

a wasting

b fasciculation

c increased tone

d flexor plantar reflex

e areflexia.

51 Which of the following is not a recognised cause of upper motor neuron weakness in the legs?

a thoracic vertebral metastasis

b cervical spondylosis

c parasagittal meningioma

d prolapsed L3/4 intervertebral disc

e multiple sclerosis.

52 Which of the following is not suggestive of an upper motor neuron lesion?

a absent abdominal reflexes

b brisk thigh adductor reflex

c absent knee jerk reflex

d brisk ankle reflex

e absent cremasteric reflex.

49 (d)

One motor neuron innervates many muscle fibres. The combination of the neuron and the fibres that it innervates is called a motor unit.

50 (c)

Lower motor neuron weakness is associated with hypotonia.

51 (d)

Prolapse of the L3/4 intervertebral disc might cause compression of the thecal sac located behind the disc space, but at this point in the vertebral column the sac contains the cauda equina, resulting in lower motor neuron signs (*note that the spinal cord terminates at the lower border of the L1 vertebral body*). A parasagittal lesion is a rare cause of upper motor neuron signs in both legs by affecting the leg areas of the motor cortices on both sides.

52 (c)

The reflex changes that occur in upper motor neuron lesions consist of exaggeration of the deep tendon reflexes and loss of superficial reflexes. In the case of the plantar reflexes, the normal flexor response is lost, releasing the extensor response.

Quick fix: Upper and lower motor neuron

	Upper motor neuron	Lower motor neuron
Site of lesion	CNS; lesion disrupts descending cerebral inputs to motor neurons in spine or brainstem	CNS or peripheral nervous system; lesion disrupts motor neuron or its axon
Wasting	Late; mild 'disuse'	Early; severe 'neurogenic'
Fasciculation	No	Yes (with fibrillation on electromyogram)
Tone	Spasticity	Hypotonia
Weakness	Yes; flexors stronger than extensors in upper limbs, extensors stronger than flexors in lower limbs	Yes; may follow distribution of single peripheral nerve(s); may be predominantly distal in polyneuropathy
Deep tendon reflexes (e.g. biceps jerk, knee jerk)	Exaggerated; ankle or patellar clonus	Absent or reduced
Superficial reflexes (e.g. abdominal reflexes)	Absent	May be absent if relevant muscles are paralysed
Plantar reflex	Extensor	Flexor, or may be absent if relevant muscles are paralysed

Nerve supply of the limbs

53 Which of the following muscles is *not* typically innervated by the ulnar nerve?

a third and fourth lumbricals

b adductor pollicis

c palmar interossei

d abductor digiti minimi

e opponens pollicis.

54 The root supply of the biceps muscle tendon reflex is principally:

a C4, C5

b C5, C6

c C6, C7

d C7, C8

e C8, T1.

55 Which muscles in the lower limb are spared in a complete proximal sciatic nerve lesion?

a hamstrings

b tibialis anterior

c soleus

d quadriceps

e extensor digitorum brevis.

56 Which of the following signs is likely to be due to a posterolateral L5/S1 disc prolapse causing unilateral left-sided S1 root compression and sciatica?

a weakness of the extensor hallucis longus

b numbness on the dorsum of the foot

c loss of the left ankle reflex

d left extensor plantar

e impaired bladder function.

53

The median nerve supplies the first and second **l**umbricals, the **o**pponens pollicis, the **a**bductor pollicis brevis and the **f**lexor pollicis brevis (= 'LOAF'). All of the other intrinsic hand muscles are supplied by the ulnar nerve. The radial nerve does not supply any intrinsic hand muscles.

54

The root supply of the biceps reflex is C5, C6. Other clinically important reflexes are the brachioradialis (C5, C6), triceps (C7, C8), knee (L,2, L3, L4) and ankle (S1, S2) jerks.

55

The sciatic nerve supplies the hamstrings, the anterior (deep peroneal nerve), lateral (superficial peroneal nerve) and posterior compartments (tibial nerve) of the calf, and the intrinsic foot muscles (tibial and deep peroneal nerves). The quadriceps muscle is supplied by the femoral nerve.

56

Left-sided S1 root compression typically causes sciatica, numbness on the sole of the foot and loss of the ankle reflex. Extensor plantar responses would suggest a lesion of the spinal cord, which is situated more rostrally within the vertebral canal. The bladder is supplied by S2–S4. The extensor hallucis longus (EHL) is supplied by the L5 nerve root.

Quick fix: Nerve supply of the limbs

	Weak muscles	Sensory loss	Reflex changes
Median nerve compression at wrist	APB, opponens pollicis	Thumb, index, middle and half of ring finger	Nil
Ulnar compression at elbow	ADM, first dorsal interosseous (DIO)	Little and half of ring finger	Nil
Radial nerve compression in upper arm	Wrist and long finger extensors	Anatomical snuffbox	Variable loss of triceps reflex
Common peroneal nerve compression at neck of fibula	Tibialis anterior, peronei	Lateral aspect of calf and dorsum of foot	Nil
C7 root	Triceps, wrist extensors	Central strip of forearm	Loss of triceps reflex
L5 root	Extensor hallucis longus	Dorsum of foot	Nil
S1 root	Gastrocnemius, soleus	Sole of foot	Loss of ankle reflex

APB, abductor pollicis brevis; ADM, abductor digiti minimi.

Sensory system

For each of questions 57–63 opposite, choose the distribution of sensory loss from the list **a** to **h** that best fits the neurological lesion described in the question.

a   loss of pain and temperature sensation in the distal limbs

b   loss of pain and temperature sensation in the left leg, and loss of proprioception and vibration sense in the right leg

c   loss of pain and temperature sensation from mid-sternum to abdomen, but preservation of light touch sensation

d   loss of all modalities of sensation on the perineum, posterior buttocks and backs of legs

e   loss of proprioception and vibration in the distal limbs

f   loss of pinprick sensation on the lateral aspect of the upper arm

g   loss of pain and temperature sensation on the left arm, trunk and leg, and on the right side of the face

h   loss of all modalities of sensation on the right side of the body.

57 Infarction in the territory of the right posterior inferior cerebellar artery.

58 Syringomyelia of the thoracic cord.

59 Small-nerve-fibre sensory neuropathy.

60 Axillary nerve damage.

61 Central L4/5 inter-vertebral disc prolapse.

62 Infarction of the left thalamus.

63 Multiple sclerosis plaque in the right side of the spinal cord at T10.

57 (g)

The ipsilateral quintothalamic tract fibres are disrupted by damage to the descending tract of the trigeminal nerve, resulting in ipsilateral loss of pain and temperature sensation on the face. The ipsilateral spinothalamic tract is also damaged – this supplies pain and temperature sensation to the opposite side of the body, fibres from the second-order neurons having decussated in the spinal cord. The medial lemniscus and principal sensory nucleus of the trigeminal nerve do not lie within the vascular territory of the posterior inferior cerebellar artery, resulting in sparing of discriminative light touch sensation on the face and proprioception and vibration sense in the limbs.

58 (c)

The expanding central cord lesion first affects the decussating spinothalamic fibres as they cross in front of the central canal to reach the contralateral tract. The fibres are laminated, with those from more rostral spinal segments lying medially. Consequently, an expanding central mass in the thoracic cord produces the sensory abnormality described – so-called 'Cuirass anaesthesia'.

59 (a)

The characteristic sensory loss of polyneuropathy occurs in a 'glove and stocking' distribution. In the case of a disease process that differentially affects small unmyelinated nerves, pain and temperature sensation will be selectively disrupted.

60

The axillary nerve supplies the skin of the 'regimental badge' region on the upper lateral arm. The nerve runs very close to the shoulder joint, and may be damaged during dislocation, resulting in this characteristic distribution of anaesthesia.

61

This type of sensory disturbance occurs in a lesion of the cauda equina affecting the lower roots (S2 and below) that lie most medially behind the lumbar intervertebral discs. Back pain, loss of bladder function and weak legs may occur in association with the sensory disturbance. This is a neurosurgical emergency – it is essential to examine sensation on the backs of the legs and buttocks in patients with acute low back pain.

62

Thalamic infarction, particularly in the sensory parts of the thalamus (ventral posterior nucleus), results in contralateral hemi-anaesthesia. This may be accompanied by extremely unpleasant burning pain (thalamic pain).

63

This is the pattern seen in the hemi-cord syndrome (Brown–Séquard). It is associated with pyramidal weakness in the ipsilateral leg and is a common consequence of multiple sclerosis, where inflammatory cord lesions tend to be patchy and incomplete.

Autonomic nervous system

64 A lesion in the Edinger–Westphal nucleus in the right midbrain would give rise to:

a impaired ipsilateral lacrimation

b loss of sweating over the ipsilateral forehead

c ipsilateral ptosis

d ipsilateral pupillary dilatation

e contralateral pupillary constriction.

65 Which of the following statements about autonomic physiology is *incorrect?*

a Sympathetic noradrenergic fibres supply cutaneous sweat glands. Their activation results in sweat production.

b Parasympathetic cholinergic fibres supply the sino-atrial node of the heart. Their activation results in bradycardia.

c Sympathetic noradrenergic fibres supply splanchnic blood vessels. Their activation results in vasoconstriction.

d Parasympathetic cholinergic fibres supply the detrusor muscle of the bladder. Their activation results in voiding.

e Sympathetic noradrenergic fibres supply the smooth muscle of the pupil. Their activation results in mydriasis.

66 Common adverse effects of pyridostigmine, an acetylcholinesterase inhibitor used in the treatment of myasthenia gravis, include:

a constipation

b tachycardia

c dry mouth

d impaired micturition

e excessive bronchial secretions.

67 Each of the following signs can be seen with Homes–Adie (tonic) pupils *except*:

a slow pupillary constriction with accommodation

b sluggish response of the pupil to 0.1% pilocarpine

c loss of deep tendon reflexes

d segmental denervation of the pupillary sphincter

e impaired pupillary constriction in response to light.

64

The Edinger–Westphal nucleus lies in the midbrain closely related to the oculomotor (III) nerve nucleus. It contains preganglionic parasympathetic neurons which supply the sphincter pupillae and ciliary muscles. Their activation results in pupillary constriction and focuses the lens for near vision.

65

The sudomotor supply to cutaneous sweat glands is derived anatomically from the sympathetic nervous system. However, unlike sympathetic postganglionic fibres elsewhere, the sudomotor fibres are cholinergic.

66

Acetylcholinesterase inhibitors give rise to side-effects suggestive of cholinergic excess. All of the symptoms listed apart from excessive bronchial secretions are more typical of a cholinergic deficit.

67

Holmes–Adie pupils are caused by degeneration of the postganglionic neurons from the ciliary ganglion innervating the sphincter pupillae. They may be associated with absent tendon reflexes. The pupillary response to light is typically absent or very delayed, with a more definite response to accommodation. The pupil constricts rapidly in response to 0.1% pilocarpine (denervation supersensitivity).

Quick fix: Causes of autonomic dysfunction

Primary

- Acute pure cholinergic dysautonomia
- Chronic pure autonomic failure
- Multiple system atrophy

Secondary

- Hereditary:
  - familial amyloid neuropathy
  - hereditary sensory and autonomic neuropathies
- Diabetes mellitus
- Guillain–Barré syndrome
- Botulism
- Lambert–Eaton syndrome
- Spinal cord transection
- Drugs, chemicals and poisons

Quick fix: Pupillary abnormalities

	Complete III nerve palsy	Horner's syndrome	Holmes–Adie pupil	Argyll Robertson pupil
Size	Dilated	Constricted	Dilated	Small, irregular
Light response	Absent	Normal	Absent	Absent
Near response (accommodation)	Absent	Normal	Slow, incomplete	Slow response
Pharmacology	Brisk constriction with 0.1% pilocarpine	Dilatation with cocaine	Brisk constriction with 0.1% pilocarpine	No response to atropine
Associated signs	Complete ptosis; weakness of superior rectus, medial rectus, inferior rectus, and inferior oblique muscles	Mild ptosis; no extra-ocular muscle weakness	Normal eye movements; no ptosis; absent tendon reflexes	Bilateral ptosis if associated with tabes dorsalis

PART 2

Investigation of neurological disease

Neuroradiology

68 Which of the following structures characteristically appears black on T2-weighted magnetic resonance imaging (MRI)?

a subcutaneous fat

b the lumen of the internal carotid artery

c grey matter of the frontal lobe

d white matter of the internal capsule

e ventricular CSF in the temporal horn of the lateral ventricle.

69 Which of the following characteristically can appear isodense with brain tissue on a non-contrast computerised tomography (CT) head scan?

a blood in acute subarachnoid haemorrhage

b intracranial air following acute head injury

c altered blood in a chronic subdural haematoma

d bone in the region adjacent to a skull fracture

e blood in an acute extradural haematoma.

70 Which of the following investigations has the highest sensitivity in the detection of berry aneurysms of the circle of Willis?

a   MR angiography

b   T2 axial MRI scan

c   CT angiography

d   T1 coronal MRI scan

e   intra-arterial angiography.

71 Which of the following features found on a CT scan is not suggestive of an acute middle cerebral artery infarct in a patient two hours after the onset of acute left hemiplegia, left homonymous hemianopia, left conjugate gaze palsy and left sensory neglect?

a   increased attenuation in the right middle cerebral artery

b   low attenuation in the head of the right caudate nucleus

c   normal CT scan

d   loss of grey matter/white matter differentiation in the right peri-sylvian ribbon

e   well-circumscribed high-attenuation area with mass effect in the right basal ganglia.

68

T2-weighted MRI shows water as white, so that the intracranial contents appear bright, with signal intensity varying according to the water content. Flowing blood appears black, so the internal carotid artery is characteristically dark.

70

Although there have been unprecedented technical advances in non-invasive imaging of the cerebral contents, diagnostic intra-arterial angiography is still the most sensitive way of detecting berry aneurysms arising from the circle of Willis.

69

The blood present acutely eventually breaks down to form fluid in a chronic subdural haematoma, which appears hypodense with respect to brain on the CT scan. At some point during this process, the blood is isodense with brain on CT and can be difficult to see, especially if the haematomas are bilateral, preventing the characteristic brain shift that may accompany a unilateral haematoma.

71

The early features of acute middle cerebral artery infarction on CT may be subtle and easily missed. A hyper-dense area with mass effect and oedema in this clinical context suggests acute haemorrhage rather than infarction.

Quick fix: Brain MRI

Things that appear bright on T1-weighted images (most pathology is dark on T1)

- Fat
- Proteinaceous fluid
- Methaemoglobin
- Melanin
- Gadolinium
- Microcalcification
- Normal vascular structures

Things that appear dark on T2-weighted images (most pathology is bright on T2)

- Air
- Minerals (dense calcification, iron, manganese)
- Blood (intracellular methaemoglobin, deoxyhaemoglobin, haemosiderin)
- Proteinaceous fluid
- Rapid vascular flow
- Melanin

EEG and evoked potentials

72 Childhood absence epilepsy is characteristically associated with the following EEG abnormalities:

a temporal lobe spike discharges

b excess frontal slow-wave activity

c 3-Hz spike and wave activity

d absent alpha rhythm

e periodic lateralised epileptiform discharges.

73 A routine normal EEG is useful for excluding the following neurological conditions:

a herpes simplex encephalitis

b Creutzfeldt–Jakob's disease

c temporal lobe epilepsy

d Alzheimer's disease

e none of the above.

74 A delayed unilateral visual evoked response (VER) is typically seen in patients with:

a corrected myopia

b retinitis pigmentosa

c anterior uveitis

d optic nerve disease

e contralateral occipital lobe lesion.

75 Which of the following statements concerning evoked responses is *incorrect*?

a Toxic optic neuropathy may be associated with an abnormal VER.

b Delayed VERs can be seen in patients with multiple sclerosis without a history of preceding visual impairment.

c Acoustic neuromas can be associated with abnormal brainstem auditory evoked responses.

d Incomplete predominantly sensory transverse myelitis can be associated with normal somatosensory evoked responses.

e Abnormal evoked responses are essential for supporting a diagnosis of multiple sclerosis.

72

Childhood absence epilepsy forms part of a group of disorders that are collectively known as the idiopathic primary generalised epilepsies (IGE). 3-Hz spike and wave activity is seen in several different IGE syndromes, and is characteristic of childhood absence epilepsy.

73

Routine EEGs are of little use in the diagnosis of neurodegenerative conditions such as Alzheimer's disease. They may also be normal in the early stages of Creutzfeldt–Jakob's disease and herpes encephalitis. Although EEGs are frequently abnormal in temporal lobe epilepsy, a normal record would not exclude the diagnosis.

74

Delayed VERs are typically seen in patients with disease that is affecting the optic nerve. They are characteristically found in optic neuritis, but may also be observed in other inflammatory and compressive optic neuropathies. Delayed VERs are not typically seen with retinal disease, glaucoma or lesions in the occipital lobe, even though vision may be profoundly affected.

75

Abnormal evoked responses are not required to make a diagnosis of clinically definite multiple sclerosis. The diagnosis rests on the demonstration of lesions affecting the central nervous system that are separated in time and space, and is supported by laboratory investigation such as MRI of the brain and spinal cord, CSF analysis for oligoclonal bands and evoked responses.

Quick fix: EEG and epilepsy

- A normal routine EEG does not exclude the diagnosis of epilepsy.
- Characteristic inter-ictal EEG abnormalities may be found in patients with idiopathic generalised epilepsy.
- Video telemetry (EEG with time-locked video recording) is of great value in distinguishing seizures from non-epileptic attacks.
- EEG localisation of seizures is essential in the preoperative assessment of patients with focal epilepsy and structural abnormalities.

Quick fix: Other syndromes associated with characteristic EEG abnormalities

- Creutzfeldt–Jakob disease (periodic sharp waves).
- Subacute sclerosing panencephalitis (periodic generalised complexes).
- Hepatic encephalopathy (bilaterally synchronous slow waves with triphasic potentials).
- Herpes simplex encephalitis (focal spike and slow-wave activity, periodic lateralised epileptiform discharges).

Lumbar puncture (LP) and cerebrospinal fluid (CSF)

76 Which of the following best describes normal cerebrospinal spinal fluid obtained by lumbar puncture, assuming that the blood glucose is 5.0 mmol/L?

a opening pressure 35 cmH$_2$O, acellular, protein 0.7 g/L, glucose 4.0 mmol/L

b opening pressure 10 cmH$_2$O, 25 lymphocytes, no red blood cells, protein 0.6 g/L, glucose 3.5 mmol/L

c opening pressure 8 cmH$_2$O, acellular, protein 0.4 g/L, glucose 3.2 mmol/L

d opening pressure 2 cmH$_2$O, acellular, protein 1.5 g/L, glucose 4.5 mmol/L

e opening pressure 12 cmH$_2$O, 100 red blood cells, 35 polymorphs, protein 1.0 g/L, glucose 1.8 mmol/L.

77 With regard to the performance of lumbar puncture:

a the procedure can only be carried out with the patient lying in the left lateral position

b use of a larger needle prevents post-lumbar-puncture headache

c palpation of the iliac crest helps to identify the L1/2 intervertebral space, which is the safest level for puncture

d venous and respiratory pressure waves may be observed in the CSF meniscus within the manometer

e aseptic technique is unnecessary, as the CNS is an immunologically privileged site.

78 Which of the following features would cast serious doubt on the diagnosis of post-lumbar puncture headache?

a   fever

b   malaise

c   vomiting

d   orthostatic head pain

e   tinnitus.

79 The presence of oligoclonal immunoglobulin bands on isoelectric focusing, which are unique to the CSF, suggests that:

a   the patient has definite multiple sclerosis

b   the blood–brain barrier has been breached

c   an infective cause of the patient's symptoms is unlikely

d   there is intrathecal synthesis of immunoglobulin

e   a laboratory artefact has given rise to a spurious result.

76

Normal CSF pressure at lumbar puncture is 5–15 cmH$_2$O. The CSF has no cells, a protein concentration of 0.15–0.6 g/L and glucose >60% blood level.

77

Lumbar puncture is performed using aseptic technique to avoid introducing infection; the patient may be lying in the left lateral position or sitting up. Palpation of the iliac crest allows identification of the L4/5 space. A smaller needle reduces the incidence of post-lumbar-puncture headache. Pressure waves may indeed be visible in the CSF meniscus within the manometer.

78

Post-lumbar-puncture low-pressure headache is typically orthostatic and associated with nausea and vomiting. In extreme circumstances, sixth nerve palsy and tinnitus have been described, but a fever should prompt a search for alternative causes of the headache.

79

Detection of oligoclonal IgG bands unique to CSF indicates intrathecal synthesis of immunoglobulin. This is consistent with multiple sclerosis in the appropriate clinical context. However, the test cannot be used to make the diagnosis alone, as various other types of CNS inflammation and some infections may be associated with the presence of oligoclonal bands.

Quick fix: Causes of CSF mononuclear pleocytosis

Infection

- Viral meningo-encephalitis (mumps, herpes simplex virus, varicella zoster virus, ECHO virus, coxsackie virus, polio virus, lymphocytic choriomeningitis, Epstein–Barr virus)
- HIV (seroconversion; chronic aseptic meningitis; asymptomatic; opportunistic infection)
- Fungal meningitis
- Atypical bacterial meningitis (Lyme borreliosis, TB, syphilis, leptospirosis, brucellosis)
- Pyogenic infection near to meninges (paranasal sinus, brain abscess)
- Partially treated pyogenic bacterial meningitis

Tumour

- Carcinoma
- Lymphoma (cells may be tumour or reactive)
- Leukaemia

Non-infective inflammation

- Multiple sclerosis
- Sarcoid
- CNS vasculitis
- Behçet's disease
- Acute disseminated encephalomyelitis

Nerve conduction studies (NCS) and electromyography (EMG)

80 Which of the following measurements is most useful for distinguishing demyelinating from axonal neuropathies?

a   compound muscle action potential amplitude

b   motor nerve conduction velocity

c   F-wave latency

d   sensory nerve action potential amplitude

e   evidence of chronic partial denervation on EMG.

81 In which of the following clinical scenarios is disposable concentric needle EMG examination most useful?

a   evaluation of inflammatory myopathy

b   excluding a significant diabetic peripheral neuropathy

c   diagnosis of steroid myopathy

d   identification of a generalised peripheral neuropathy

e   diagnosis of generalised myasthenia gravis.

82 Which of the following abnormalities would *not* be expected in right carpal tunnel syndrome?

a reduced amplitude of the compound muscle action potential (CMAP) in the right abductor pollicis brevis (APB)

b prolonged right APB distal motor latency

c absent sensory action potential from right index finger with measurement at the wrist (F2-w)

d prolonged right abductor digiti minimi (ADM) distal motor latency

e prolonged right index finger to wrist sensory nerve action potential (SNAP) latency.

83 Abnormal single-fibre EMG is seen frequently in all of the following neurological disorders *except*:

a myasthenia gravis

b Lambert–Eaton myasthenic syndrome

c congenital myasthenic syndromes

d chronic inflammatory demyelinating polyneuropathy

e botulism.

80

Nerve conduction studies are particularly useful for discriminating between demyelinating and axonal neuropathies. The motor conduction velocities are slower in demyelinating neuropathies, with a cut-off value of 39 m/s in the upper limb and 35 m/s in the lower limb.

81

EMG is of little value in the assessment of neuropathy, where nerve conduction studies are of particular use, other than to document whether there has been axonal degeneration and thus denervation. EMG is also of limited value in the assessment of metabolic and steroid-induced myopathies. Inflammatory myopathies are typically associated with an abnormal EMG with short duration, polyphasic, small motor unit potentials, positive sharp waves and occasionally fibrillations.

82

Carpal tunnel syndrome (compression of the median nerve at the wrist) classically presents with nocturnal pain and paraesthesiae which may be poorly localised and spread to involve the forearm. Nerve conduction studies are helpful, typically showing delayed or absent sensory action potentials from median nerve innervated digits, delayed distal motor latency to the APB and occasionally, if severe, a small CMAP from the APB. The condition is typically bilateral, which explains why asymptomatic neurophysiological changes may be found in the other hand. The ADM muscle is supplied by the ulnar nerve, so is not affected by median nerve compression.

83

Single-fibre EMG is an extremely sensitive technique for the diagnosis of disorders that affect neuromuscular transmission. However, abnormalities are not specific for a single disorder, and may be seen in myasthenia gravis as well as congenital myasthenic syndromes, the Lambert–Eaton syndrome and botulism.

Quick fix: Nerve conduction studies in neuropathy

	Demyelinating neuropathy	Axonal neuropathy
Compound muscle action potential	Dispersion of potential	Reduced amplitude
Sensory nerve action potential	Absent	Absent
Distal motor latency	Prolonged	Normal
Motor conduction velocities	Reduced: <39 m/s in arms and <35 m/s in legs	Normal

Quick fix: Neurogenic and myopathic EMG

	Denervation	Myositis
Spontaneous activity	+++	+
Duration of motor unit potential	Increased	Normal or decreased
Size of motor unit potential	Increased	Decreased
Polyphasic potentials	Yes	Yes
Interference pattern	Reduced	Normal/full

PART 3

Diseases of the nervous system

Cerebrovascular disease I

84 In an infarction involving the entire territory supplied by the left middle cerebral artery (MCA), typically:

a there is hemiparesis with sparing of the face, as the face area of the motor cortex is supplied by the anterior cerebral artery

b there is a homonymous upper quadrantanopia, as the segment of the optic radiation within the temporal lobe is supplied by the posterior circulation

c it is unusual for brain oedema to present a problem, as the infarcted tissue rapidly involutes

d there may be paralysis of conjugate gaze to the contralateral side

e aphasia is uncommon; Wernicke's area is not supplied by the MCA.

85 All of the following are characteristic features of posterior inferior cerebellar artery occlusion *except*:

a vertigo

b vomiting

c ipsilateral dysmetria

d contralateral pyramidal signs

e ipsilateral Horner's syndrome.

86 All of the following are recognised causes of cerebral arterial infarction *except*:

a neurosyphilis

b marantic endocarditis

c thrombotic thrombocytopenic purpura

d factor IX deficiency

e Takayasu's disease.

87 Which of the following statements best describes the management of carotid stenosis?

a symptomatic stenosis of 70–99% should be managed by endarterectomy

b symptomatic stenosis of 50–99% should be managed by warfarin and aspirin in combination

c symptomatic stenosis of 30–100% should be managed by endarterectomy and warfarin

d asymptomatic stenosis of all grades should be managed by endarterectomy

e asymptomatic stenosis of 100% requires emergency endarterectomy and heparin.

84 (d)

Left middle cerebral territory infarction typically causes right hemiparesis (face and arm worse than leg), dysphasia, right conjugate gaze palsy and right homonymous hemianopia or inferior quadrantanopia. There may be significant mass effect from oedema, especially in younger patients.

85 (d)

The pyramidal tracts lie medially within the pyramids of the medulla, and are therefore outside the vascular territory of the posterior inferior cerebellar artery.

86 (d)

All of the listed diseases are prothrombotic states that have been associated with ischaemic stroke, apart from factor IX deficiency, which is an inherited haemophilia associated with intracranial haemorrhage.

87 (a)

Clinical trials support the use of early (up to 6 months) carotid endarterectomy in the management of patients with transient ischaemic attack and an ipsilateral internal carotid artery stenosis of 70–99%. Warfarin is of no proven benefit in the management of carotid stenosis. Complete occlusion of the carotid artery reduces the risk of embolism, so surgery is usually avoided unless there are severe problems on the other side.
At present there is no good evidence to recommend the use of surgery for asymptomatic stenosis.

facts fixed on Cerebrovascular disease I

Quick fix: Cerebral infarct syndromes

Syndrome	Clinical features	Dead or dependent at 6 months	Vascular territory
Total anterior circulation infarct (TACI)	(i) weakness of the whole of one side of the body *and* (ii) homonymous hemianopia *and* (iii) focal cognitive deficit (e.g. aphasia, neglect)	95%	ICA; proximal MCA
Partial anterior circulation infarct (PACI)	(i) two of the three features of TACI *or* (ii) isolated cognitive deficit *or* (iii) isolated proprioceptive deficit. Sensory/motor deficit may involve only one limb	45%	Branch MCA or ACA, or boundary-zone ischaemia
Lacunar anterior circulation infarct (LACI)	(i) pure motor disturbance *or* (ii) pure sensory loss (not isolated proprioceptive loss – see PACI) *or* (iii) other focal non-cortical deficit	35%	Small penetrating arteries
Posterior circulation infarct (PoCI)	(i) brainstem signs *or* (ii) cerebellar signs *or* (iii) homonymous hemianopia/cortical blindness	30%	Vertebro-basilar system or PCA

MCA, middle cerebral artery; ACA, anterior cerebral artery; PCA, posterior cerebral artery; ICA, internal carotid artery.

Cerebrovascular disease II

88 Which of the following cutaneous signs is *least* likely to be relevant in explaining the aetiology of an ischaemic stroke?

a livedo reticularis

b nicotine-stained fingers

c necrobiosis lipoidica

d heliotrope rash and nail-fold telangiectasia

e Osler's nodes and Janeway lesions.

89 With regard to the treatment of acute ischaemic stroke, which of the following statements is true?

a Aspirin should be given after a delay of 14 days to reduce the haemorrhagic risk.

b Heparin is mandatory to prevent deep venous thrombosis in immobile stroke patients.

c In cases of non-rheumatic atrial fibrillation associated with stroke, warfarin should be commenced as soon as possible after admission.

d Aggressive treatment of raised blood pressure improves the prognosis.

e Early attention to nutrition is important.

90 With regard to the differentiation of primary intracerebral haemorrhage from ischaemic infarct in patients presenting with stroke, which of the following statements is true?

a Headache strongly suggests the presence of haemorrhage.

b Early coma excludes infarct.

c It is not possible to distinguish a haemorrhage from an infarct clinically.

d The sites of typical haemorrhage and infarct give rise to characteristic patterns of deficit.

e Blood seen on the CT scan is always caused by primary intracerebral haemorrhage.

91 Following a cerebellar hemisphere infarct, which of the following statements is true?

a The anatomical diagnosis will usually be clear because of obvious cerebellar signs.

b Early discharge from hospital is advisable to encourage ambulation and functional recovery.

c Deterioration following the infarct usually indicates propagating thrombus in the arterial system and carries a poor prognosis.

d Vomiting is unusual because the vomiting reflexes are co-ordinated and regulated in other areas of the brain.

e Fourth ventricular obstruction is a common and treatable complication.

88

Heliotrope rash and nail-fold telangiectasia are characteristic of dermatomyositis, which is not associated with ischaemic stroke. The other cutaneous signs are associated with underlying conditions that predispose to cerebral infarction (livedo reticularis – antiphospholipid antibody syndrome; nicotine-stained fingers – atheroma; necrobiosis lipoidica – diabetes mellitus; Osler's nodes and Janeway lesions – infective endocarditis).

89

Nutrition is often overlooked in stroke patients, especially when there are difficulties with swallowing or impairment of motivation or motor function. Aspirin should be started immediately after ischaemic stroke. Heparin is harmful and should be avoided. Warfarin is usually commenced after a delay of 10–14 days in cases of atrial fibrillation associated with stroke, to reduce the likelihood of secondary haemorrhage. Hypertension occurring after cerebral infarct is part of a compensatory response, and its aggressive acute treatment may exacerbate the ischaemia without having any significant effect on secondary prevention.

90

It is not possible to distinguish haemorrhage and infarct clinically with any reliability. All stroke patients should undergo brain imaging.

91

Cerebellar hemisphere stroke does not always produce the expected ipsilateral cerebellar signs, even when the infarct is large. Secondary oedema may cause compression of the fourth ventricle with obstructive hydrocephalus over the 24–48 hours after the infarct. It is very important to observe patients with this condition so that appropriate therapy can be instituted if this complication arises. Vertigo and vomiting are common in cerebellar infarction.

Quick fix: Causes of ischaemic stroke

Atheromatous thrombo-embolism (50%)

Intracranial small-vessel disease (25%)

Cardiac embolism (20%)

- Atrial fibrillation
- Atrial myxoma
- Infective endocarditis
- Rheumatic endocarditis
- Prosthetic heart valve
- Acute myocardial infarction
- Dilated cardiomyopathy

Rare causes (< 5%)

- Arterial dissection
- Antiphospholipid syndrome
- Giant-cell arteritis
- Drugs (cocaine, amphetamine)

Very rare causes (< 1%)

- Other vasculitides
- Vascular malformations and aneurysms
- Unusual embolism (fat, fibrocartilage)
- Haematological disorders (polycythaemia, thrombocythaemia, thrombotic thrombocytopenic purpura, leukaemia, paroxysmal nocturnal haemoglobinuria, hyperviscosity, hereditary thrombophilia)
- Cancer
- Migraine
- Inherited metabolic diseases (mitochondrial encephalomyopathy with lactic acidosis and stroke-like episodes – MELAS; homocystinuria)
- Pregnancy/oestrogens

Subarachnoid haemorrhage

92 A patient is admitted to the Accident and Emergency department with severe headache and photophobia. All of the following features are consistent with a diagnosis of spontaneous subarachnoid haemorrhage, secondary to a ruptured saccular aneurysm of the circle of Willis, *except*:

a   a temperature of 37.8°C

b   subhyaloid haemorrhage

c   nuchal rigidity

d   widespread purpuric rash

e   anterior T-wave inversion on the ECG.

93 With regard to the investigation of subarachnoid haemorrhage, which of the following statements is true?

a   A CT scan should be delayed, to allow diagnostic features to develop.

b   Arterial cerebral angiography is the 'gold standard'; it will show a berry aneurysm in all cases.

c   A contrast-enhanced CT scan improves the diagnostic sensitivity.

d   Lumbar puncture is dangerous and should be avoided.

e   A CT scan can be normal in up to 10% of cases.

94 A patient suffers a subarachnoid haemorrhage secondary to rupture of an intracranial aneurysm. She is fully conscious initially, but becomes unresponsive 24 hours later. The following are characteristic causes of deterioration following a subarachnoid haemorrhage *except*:

a hypernatraemia secondary to the syndrome of inappropriate antidiuretic hormone secretion (SIADH)

b cerebral vasospasm

c drug intoxication

d communicating hydrocephalus

e hypoxaemia secondary to neurogenic pulmonary oedema.

95 With regard to the cerebrospinal fluid obtained by lumbar puncture from a patient with suspected subarachnoid haemorrhage, which of the following statements is true?

a The appearance of red blood cells can be ignored, as it is usually attributable to a traumatic tap.

b The opening pressure may be elevated.

c Xanthochromia appears immediately after the clinical ictus.

d The appearance of any white cells should cast doubt on the diagnosis.

e The protein concentration is not usually elevated.

92

A purpuric rash should immediately alert the physician to the possibility of meningococcal meningitis and septicaemia in this clinical setting, prompting the withdrawal of blood for culture and the administration of high-dose intravenous antibiotics without delay. The other features are compatible with subarachnoid haemorrhage.

93

CT can be normal after SAH; the diagnostic yield falls rapidly with time after clinical ictus, so the earlier the scan is performed the better. Acute blood on CT has high attenuation and is easier to see on a non-contrast scan. It is essential to perform lumbar puncture in cases where SAH is clinically possible and the CT scan normal, because 5–10% of patients with SAH have a normal CT. The characteristic CSF finding of xanthochromia (yellow discolouration of the CSF supernatant due to accumulation of the haemoglobin metabolite bilirubin) takes 12 hours to appear in the CSF, so the lumbar puncture should be delayed until 12–24 hours post-ictus. Angiography might not show any abnormality, depending on the cause of the bleeding.

94

SIADH may follow an acute intracerebral event such as subarachnoid haemorrhage, and causes *hypo*natraemia rather than *hyper*natraemia. The other items are characteristic causes of clinical deterioration following a subarachnoid haemorrhage.

95

The characteristic findings in the CSF of a patient with SAH are raised opening pressure, bloodstained CSF with numerous red blood cells, xanthrochromic supernatant and raised protein levels. Xanthochromia does not appear until 12–24 hours after the SAH, by which time there may also be an inflammatory reaction to the presence of blood in the CSF, leading to a higher WBC/RBC ratio than would be expected from the peripheral blood count.

Quick fix: Causes of spontaneous subarachnoid haemorrhage

- Ruptured aneurysm of circle of Willis (85%)
- Idiopathic perimesencephalic haemorrhage (10%)
- Rare causes (5%):
  - arteriovenous malformation of brain or spine
  - arterial dissection
  - cerebral vasculitis (polyarteritis nodosa – PAN, primary CNS angiitis)
  - mycotic aneurysm
  - pituitary apoplexy
  - drugs (cocaine, anticoagulants)

Quick fix: Reasons for clinical deterioration within hours to days after subarachnoid haemorrhage

- Rebleed
- Vasospasm
- Hydrocephalus
- Drugs (especially opiate analgesics)
- Hypoxia (neurogenic pulmonary oedema)
- Hyponatraemia
- Seizures

Venous sinus thrombosis

96 All of the following are recognised causes of sagittal sinus thrombosis *except*:

a   inflammatory bowel disease

b   pregnancy and the puerperium

c   systemic malignancy

d   viral meningitis

e   septicaemia.

97 Which of the following best describes the clinical signs of cavernous sinus thrombosis?

a   painful red eye, papilloedema and lesions of cranial nerves III, V and VII

b   pulsatile proptosis, papilloedema and lesions of cranial nerves III, IV and V

c   non-reducible proptosis, papilloedema and lesions of cranial nerves III, IV and VII

d   painless proptosis, papilloedema and lesions of cranial nerves II, III and V

e   pain, proptosis, papilloedema and lesions of cranial nerves III, IV, V and VI.

98 Which of the following statements is true with regard to the treatment of sagittal sinus thrombosis?

a The presence of haemorrhagic changes on the CT scan absolutely contraindicates the use of anticoagulants.

b Changes in intracranial pressure are small and do not usually require treatment.

c Heparin worsens the prognosis and should not be used.

d Focal or generalised seizures are common and require anticonvulsant treatment.

e Warfarin is the only treatment that has been shown to improve outcome.

99 Which of the following best describes the CSF findings at lumbar puncture in idiopathic thrombosis of the right lateral sinus (assume a blood glucose concentration of 5.1 mmol/L)?

a opening pressure 27 cmH$_2$O, no cells, protein 2.0 g/L, glucose 3.0 mmol/L

b opening pressure 10 cmH$_2$O, 200 red blood cells, protein 0.5 g/L, glucose 3.0 mmol/L

c opening pressure 27 cmH$_2$O, no cells, protein 0.9 g/L, glucose 3.0 mmol/L

d opening pressure 10 cmH$_2$O, 30 lymphocytes, protein 1.8 g/L, glucose 0.5 mmol/L

e opening pressure 27cmH$_2$O, 30 lymphocytes, protein 1.3 g/L, glucose 3.0 mmol/L.

96

Viral meningitis is a self-limiting condition that is not associated with cerebral venous sinus thrombosis. The remaining systemic conditions are all recognised associations of venous sinus thrombosis.

97

Cavernous sinus thrombosis is painful and characterised by lesions of the cranial nerves that traverse the sinus (VI) or its wall (III, IV and Va) in addition to signs of orbital venous hypertension (papilloedema, chemosis, exophthalmos).

98

The treatment of sagittal sinus thrombosis is largely supportive, with treatment of raised intracranial pressure and seizures forming an important part. There is debate over the role of heparin. There have been two randomised clinical trials, and a recent Cochrane review of these concluded that heparin was safe (probably even if there is haemorrhage on the CT scan), but that evidence of efficacy was not conclusive. On this basis, many clinicians treat the condition with intravenous heparin.

99

In the absence of local meningeal disease or extension of middle-ear sepsis into the cranium, the CSF in lateral sinus thrombosis usually shows mild elevation of protein concentration, but no cells. However, the pressure is raised, as the thrombosis causes intracranial venous hypertension, with secondary failure of CSF reabsorption.

Quick fix: Clinical syndromes of intracranial venous thrombosis

- *Sagittal sinus* – headache, papilloedema, focal seizures, leg weakness
- *Cavernous sinus* – pain, proptosis, chemosis, papilloedema, cranial nerve lesions (III, IV, Va and VI)
- *Lateral sinus* – headache, papilloedema (often following middle-ear sepsis – 'otitic hydrocephalus')
- *Deep venous system (vein of Galen and internal cerebral veins)* – headache, early coma, signs of upper brainstem and diencephalic infarction

Quick fix: Causes of intracranial venous thrombosis

- *Pregnancy and the puerperium*
- *Dehydration*
- *Haematological disease* – thrombocythaemia, polycythaemia, paroxysmal nocturnal haemoglobinuria, sickle-cell disease, hereditary coagulopathies
- *Systemic disease* – malignancy, systemic lupus erythematosus and antiphospholipid syndrome, nephrotic syndrome, inflammatory bowel disease, Behçet's disease
- *Drugs* – combined oral contraceptive, androgens, ecstasy
- *Local pathology* – otitis, sinusitis, dental abscess, tonsillitis, tumour, chronic meningitis, subdural empyema
- *Idiopathic* (20%)

Head injury

100 Early epileptic seizures following a head injury are more likely if any of the following features are present *except*:

a depressed skull fracture

b blunt cranial trauma

c intracranial haematoma

d prolonged post-traumatic amnesia (> 24 hours)

e injury in a young child.

101 Which of the following clinical features would cast doubt on a diagnosis of benign post-traumatic headache 2 months after a head injury?

a irritability

b fatigue

c light-headedness

d severe headache

e disorientation.

102 Which of the following statements is true regarding chronic subdural haematoma (SDH)?

a   A fluctuating cognitive deficit may be the only clinical abnormality.

b   A clear history of head injury is apparent in most cases.

c   Papilloedema is usually present, suggesting that the intracranial pressure is raised.

d   Chronic SDH characteristically affects younger patients.

e   Bilateral SDH is extremely rare.

103 Which of the following statements is true regarding extradural haematoma?

a   The characteristic syndrome may evolve slowly over a period of several weeks.

b   The source of blood is often branches of the middle meningeal artery.

c   Urgent evacuation of the haematoma is unnecessary, as the blood is extradural and thus unlikely to compromise cerebral function.

d   A unilateral fixed and dilated pupil is often seen contralateral to the haematoma.

e   CT scanning is diagnostically unhelpful, because the thin layer of blood is difficult to distinguish from overlying bone.

100

Blunt trauma is associated with a reduced risk of post-traumatic epilepsy compared with a penetrating injury. The other listed options are all risk factors for epilepsy after head injury.

101

After minor head injury, it is common to observe headache in association with mild, non-specific deficits in cognition (e.g. poor concentration), fatigue and irritability. However, frank disorientation should raise the suspicion that there is another diagnosis (intracranial haematoma, hydrocephalus), or that the injury was much more severe than was previously thought.

102

Chronic subdural haematoma is more common in patients with cerebral atrophy and those with blood-clotting abnormalities. Such patients are often elderly, alcoholic or taking antiplatelet or anticoagulant drugs. Focal signs may be absent, as may be signs of raised intracranial pressure. Frequently no past history of head injury can be elicited. Chronic subdural haematoma may be bilateral.

103

Acute extradural haematoma characteristically occurs several hours after a significant head injury. Arterial blood, often from the middle meningeal artery or its branches, collects between the dura and the skull, stripping the meninges away from the bone. This results in the classical convex-shaped high-density lesion on CT scanning. Urgent neurosurgical intervention is needed to prevent displacement of the temporal lobe through the tentorial hiatus, with secondary brainstem compression and death. The third cranial nerve may be compressed by the herniated temporal lobe, resulting initially in an ipsilateral dilated fixed pupil, followed by a complete third nerve palsy.

Epilepsy I

104 All of the following types of epileptic phenomena suggest that seizures originate in the stated areas of the cortex *except*:

a simple stereotyped visual hallucinations – occipital lobe

b complex stereotyped visual hallucinations – inferior temporal lobe

c stereotyped olfactory hallucinations – uncus of the temporal lobe

d complex stereotyped left-arm posturing – right frontal lobe

e conjugate deviation of the eyes to the left – left frontal lobe.

105 With regard to the investigation of an adult who has suffered a single seizure, which of the following statements is true?

a Imaging is unnecessary if there are no focal signs.

b Imaging is essential, and CT is the modality of choice.

c Imaging is unnecessary if there was not a focal aura.

d Imaging is usually required, and MRI is the modality of choice.

e Imaging should be delayed until a second seizure occurs.

106 With regard to the first aid of someone who is having a generalised tonic–clonic convulsion, which of the following statements is true?

a It is mandatory to prevent the patient from biting his tongue.

b If at all possible, intravenous benzodiazepine should be given.

c Prevention of injury by removing sharp or hot objects from the immediate vicinity of the patient is an important measure.

d A pharyngeal airway should be inserted to prevent hypoxia.

e Acute rhabdomyolysis should be prevented by restraining the patient.

107 Which of the following features suggests that an attack of altered consciousness was epileptic rather than syncopal?

a prolonged amnesia after the attack

b a few asynchronous twitching movements in the limbs during the attack

c nausea and vomiting on recovery

d the attack being preceded by an aura of vision closing in and hearing fading

e profuse sweating during the attack.

104

Epileptic activity in the region of the frontal eye fields on the left would be expected to drive conjugate deviation of the eyes towards the right. The other regions are correctly associated with clinical seizure types.

105

The answer to this question has changed with the availability and accessibility of non-invasive methods of imaging without exposure to X-rays. After a single seizure with no residual focal signs, the diagnostic yield from imaging is not very high, especially if there is an identifiable precipitant such as alcohol or drugs of abuse. However, a treatable lesion might be found, such as a benign tumour, so most adults who have a seizure should undergo MRI scanning.

106

Most generalised seizures are self-limiting and do not require acute pharmacological intervention. The patient should be protected from harm by making the immediate environment safe, and by lying the patient on their side to help to protect the airway. Other measures, such as restraint, trying to insert an oropharyngeal airway or preventing the patient from biting their tongue, are likely to result in injury to the patient or the first-aid giver, and should therefore be avoided.

107

Distinguishing an epileptic event from a syncopal event can be difficult. A few jerks or twitches are not uncommon in syncope. Nausea and vomiting are more common in syncope than in epilepsy, as is the hypotensive aura of fading vision and hearing and the compensatory sympathetic over-activity that results in pallor and sweating. However, prolonged amnesia after the attack is very unusual in syncope. This symptom would strongly suggest that the attack was epileptic in the right clinical context.

Quick fix: Proposed new International League Against Epilepsy (ILAE) classification of epileptic seizure types (2001)

Self-limited seizure types

Generalised seizures
- Tonic–clonic seizures (includes variations beginning with a clonic phase)
- Absence seizures (typical, atypical and myoclonic)
- Tonic seizures
- Atonic seizures

Focal seizures
- Focal sensory seizures:
  - with elementary sensory symptoms
  - with experiential sensory symptoms
- Focal motor seizures:
  - with elementary clonic motor signs
  - with asymmetrical tonic motor signs
  - with typical (temporal lobe) automatisms
- Secondarily generalised seizures

Continuous seizure types

Generalised status epilepticus
- Generalised tonic–clonic status epilepticus
- Absence status epilepticus

Focal status epilepticus
- Epilepsia partialis continua
- Aura continua
- Limbic status epilepticus (psychomotor status)

Epilepsy II

108 Which of the following statements about the measurement of blood levels of anticonvulsant drugs is true?

a It is not possible to measure the lamotrigine blood level.

b Phenytoin levels can be useful, as the metabolism of this drug is non-linear.

c Sodium valproate blood levels correlate well with therapeutic efficacy.

d The carbamazepine blood level may be used to exclude toxicity.

e Sodium valproate blood levels correlate well with toxicity.

109 Which of the following statements best describes a clinically important interaction between anticonvulsant drugs?

a Carbamazepine induces the metabolism of gabapentin.

b Sodium valproate inhibits the metabolism of lamotrigine.

c Phenytoin inhibits the metabolism of sodium valproate.

d Levetiracetam displaces gabapentin from binding sites on albumin.

e Topiramate blocks the renal excretion of sodium valproate.

Match the drugs listed below to the indications in questions 110–116:

a   lamotrigine

b   topiramate

c   sodium valproate

d   carbamazepine

e   vigabatrin

f   gabapentin

g   phenobarbitone.

110   A 16-year-old boy with generalised seizures, absences and myoclonic jerks on waking.

111   Infantile spasms.

112   Childhood typical absences ('petit mal').

113   Acute treatment of status epilepticus, if benzodiazepines are unhelpful.

114   Licensed treatment of trigeminal neuralgia if carbamazepine is not tolerated.

115   Proven efficacy as an anti-migrainous prophylactic.

116   Treatment of primary generalised epilepsy in a 17-year-old girl.

108

It is possible to measure blood levels of most drugs, but only a few are helpful clinically. Phenytoin levels are often helpful, because the metabolism of the drug saturates at blood levels just above the therapeutic level, resulting in toxicity. In addition, there are many other drugs that affect the pharmacokinetics of phenytoin. Sodium valproate blood levels do not correlate well with tissue levels, therapeutic effect or toxicity. The therapeutic range for carbamazepine does not necessarily apply to all patients, and dose-limiting side-effects can be encountered well within the therapeutic range.

109

This is very important. The dose of lamotrigine must be at least halved and the drug introduced very slowly if it is to be added to sodium valproate therapy. Failure to adhere to this may result in acute toxicity (dizziness, unsteadiness) and rash (including erythema multiforme and Stevens–Johnson's syndrome). The remaining 'interactions' are fictional.

110

Valproate is the drug of choice for primary generalised epilepsy in most instances. In young women of childbearing age, many advocate the use of lamotrigine because of the teratogenic potential of valproate. In this particular case, the diagnosis is most likely to be juvenile myoclonic epilepsy (JME), which can be worsened considerably by treatment with carbamazepine. Valproate is most definitely the drug of first choice here.

111

Vigabatrin has become an alternative to adrenocorticotropic hormone (ACTH) therapy for infantile spasms. It is not yet known which treatment is more effective.

112

See question 110. Ethosuximide is an alternative.

113

Intravenous phenobarbitone (10 mg/kg) is a useful and effective drug for the acute treatment of status epilepticus, when initial treatment with intravenous benzodiazepine has failed to terminate seizure activity. Intravenous phenytoin (15–18 mg/kg) is an alternative.

114 (f)

Gabapentin is an effective treatment for trigeminal neuralgia and other types of neurogenic pain. At present its use in trigeminal neuralgia is mainly to treat patients who do not tolerate or respond to carbamazepine.

115 (c)

There is good evidence that valproate is efficacious in preventing migraine attacks.

116 (a)

See question 110. Although valproate would be a good choice for treating the epileptic syndrome, in this case (i) the possibility of the patient becoming pregnant while taking a proven teratogen, (ii) the potential for weight gain and hair loss as potential side-effects and (iii) a possible aetiologic relationship between valproate and polycystic ovaries means that valproate is an unsuitable drug for this patient; lamotrigine is the most suitable alternative from the list given.

Quick fix: Driving and epilepsy in the UK

- Following an epileptic seizure, patients must not drive and must contact the DVLA.
- The law does not recognise any distinction between focal and generalised seizures.
- For private car and motorcycle license ('group 1'):
  - a year must elapse following a seizure (on or off medication) before driving may be resumed
  - if seizures continue only during sleep, then driving may recommence 3 years after the last attack that occurred during wakefulness
  - if medication is withdrawn, the patient must not drive from the time when medication is reduced until 6 months after stopping medication completely.
- For heavy goods and bus license ('group 2'):
  - 10 years must elapse off medication, without seizures, before driving may be resumed.
- Provoked seizures (other than those caused by alcohol or illicit drugs) may be dealt with on an individual basis.

Parkinson's disease and akinetic–rigid syndromes I

117 Which of the following physical signs is suggestive of parkinsonism?

a paresis

b bradycardia

c hypomimia

d ataxia

e spasticity.

118 Which of the following features would cast doubt on the diagnosis of Parkinson's disease?

a up-gaze paresis in an elderly patient

b failure to improve after 150 mg of L-dopa daily

c strictly unilateral signs at onset

d constipation and urinary urgency

e jerky, irregular tremor and stimulus-sensitive myoclonus.

119 Which of the following statements is true regarding the pathology of diseases associated with an akinetic–rigid syndrome?

a The hallmark pathological change of Parkinson's disease is the neuronal intranuclear inclusion, the Lewy body.

b Globose tangles are seen within substantia nigra pigmented neurons in progressive supranuclear palsy.

c The pathology of multiple system atrophy is dominated by cell loss without characteristic inclusion bodies.

d The major pathological changes of corticobasal degeneration occur within the occipital lobe of the brain.

e Infarction of the putamen is a characteristic finding in carbon monoxide poisoning.

120 Which of the following drugs is not a recognised cause of secondary parkinsonism?

a carbamazepine

b metoclopramide

c fluoxetine

d phenytoin

e nifedipine.

117 (c)

Hypomimia refers to a lack of spontaneous facial expression, and is a manifestation of akinesia (loss of spontaneous and associated movement) typical of parkinsonism. Other signs might include bradykinesia (slowness of movement), tremor, rigidity, falls and non-motor manifestations. Loss of strength (paresis – upper or lower motor neuron) is not a feature, and neither are ataxia and dysdiadochokinesis (cerebellar disease).

118 (e)

Jerky postural tremor and stimulus-sensitive myoclonus are more typical of multiple system atrophy (MSA), than idiopathic Parkinson's disease (PD), although distinguishing early PD from early MSA can be extremely difficult clinically. Other features that might suggest MSA include failure of L-dopa treatment at an adequate dose (> 600–1000 mg/24 hours) for an adequate length of time (> 3 months), symmetrical onset, cerebellar signs or autonomic failure (however, urinary urgency is common in PD, and constipation is almost universal). Some restriction of up-gaze is common in elderly patients. However, slow vertical saccades and severe early down-gaze paresis in a patient with Parkinsonism, would suggest progressive supranuclear palsy rather than PD.

119 (b)

The Lewy body is a neuronal *cytoplasmic* inclusion body that is the hallmark of Parkinson's disease, and is immunoreactive for α-synuclein. MSA is associated with *glial* cytoplasmic inclusions that are also immunoreactive for α-synuclein, but which have a different morphology to Lewy bodies. Progressive supranuclear palsy is characterised by globose tangles that are immunoreactive for microtubule-associated protein tau. Corticobasal degeneration (CBD) is also associated with tau-positive neuronal inclusions, but the distribution of the pathology is very different, CBD being particularly associated with pathological changes in the frontal lobe of the brain. Carbon monoxide poisoning characteristically produces infarction of the globus pallidus, resulting in a parkinsonian state.

120

Carbamazepine has not been reported to cause parkinsonism. The other drugs are all recognised causes of an akinetic–rigid syndrome, and an accurate drug history is an important part of the assessment of a patient with possible Parkinson's disease.

Quick fix: Causes of parkinsonism

- Sporadic late-onset neurodegenerative diseases:
  - Parkinson's disease (PD)
  - multiple system atrophy (MSA)
  - progressive supranuclear palsy (PSP)
  - corticobasal degeneration (CBD)
- Drugs (neuroleptics, anti-emetics, lithium, calcium-channel blockers, phenytoin, selective serotonin reuptake inhibitors)
- Toxins (1-methyl-4-phenyl-1,2,3,6-tetrahydropyridine – MPTP, carbon monoxide, paraquat, cyanide, alcohol withdrawal, manganese)
- Genetic neurodegenerative diseases (Wilson's disease, juvenile-onset Huntington's disease, Hallervorden–Spatz disease, more than 40 other rare syndromes associated with parkinsonism)
- Encephalitis (after infection or rarely acute infection)
- Metabolic (post-hypoxic, mitochondrial disease)

Parkinson's disease and akinetic–rigid syndromes II

121 Which of the following diseases is not a recognised cause of a parkinsonian gait?

a multiple system atrophy

b hypothyroidism

c subfrontal meningioma

d Huntington's disease

e colloid cyst of third ventricle.

122 With regard to the treatment of early Parkinson's disease, which of the following statements is true?

a Early use of L-dopa is unwise, because the drug is highly toxic to the substantia nigra and accelerates the rate of clinical decline.

b Early use of dopamine agonists is protective against the development of motor fluctuations.

c Early avoidance of L-dopa may delay the onset of dyskinesia.

d Modern dopamine agonists are as good a symptomatic treatment as L-dopa.

e Selegiline slows the rate of clinical progression and should usually be prescribed to most patients with Parkinson's disease.

In questions 123–128, match the drug to the mode of action listed below:

a   inhibitor of catechol-O-methyl transferase

b   agonist at D_1 and D_2 dopamine receptors

c   inhibitor of monoamine oxidase B

d   antagonist at cholinergic muscarinic receptors

e   peripheral dopa decarboxylase inhibitor

f   antagonist at n-methyl-D-aspartate (NMDA) receptors.

123 Ropinirole.

124 Selegiline.

125 Entacapone.

126 Benserazide.

127 Cabergoline.

128 Amantadine.

129 Which of the following is not a recognised non-motor complication of Parkinson's disease?

a   hyperphagia

b   REM-sleep behaviour disorder

c   dementia

d   urinary urgency

e   depression out of proportion to the degree of physical disability.

121 (b)

Predominant 'lower body parkinsonism', the presence of a shuffling gait without other signs of Parkinson's disease, may be caused by a number of diseases, including benign tumours, cerebrovascular disease and hydrocephalus. Multiple system atrophy is a well-recognised cause of parkinsonism, as is the juvenile-onset form of Huntington's disease ('Westphal variant'). Hypothyroidism does cause general slowing, but gait disorders are unusual and attributable to neuropathy, myopathy or rarely a cerebellar syndrome.

122 (c)

Trials suggest that the onset of L-dopa induced dyskinesias in PD may be delayed by early use of dopaminergic agonists instead of L-dopa, but this is usually at the expense of less satisfactory symptom control, as the dopamine agonists are less efficacious than L-dopa. There is no firm evidence to support any of the following assertions: (i) that dopaminergic agonists or selegiline slow the rate of clinical decline; (ii) that L-dopa increases the rate of clinical decline in PD; or (iii) that dopaminergic agonists protect against the later emergence of dyskinesia once L-dopa is introduced.

123 (b)

124 (c)

125 (a)

126 (e)

127 (b)

128 (f)

Amantadine was originally developed as an antiviral compound, but is also helpful for treating some symptoms of Parkinson's disease, including gait freezing and L-dopa induced dyskinesias. It has a number of pharmacological actions, one of which is to antagonise the actions of glutamate at NMDA type excitatory amino acid receptors.

129 (a)

Hyperphagia is not a recognised feature of Parkinson's disease, but may follow hypothalamic or bilateral temporal lobe damage. The other listed features are all well-recognised non-motor manifestations of Parkinson's disease. Depression is very important, as it accounts for much of the disability of Parkinson's disease and is treatable.

Quick fix: Non-motor manifestations of Parkinson's disease

Autonomic manifestations

- Constipation
- Detrusor hyper-reflexia
- Impotence
- Postural hypotension

Psychiatric manifestations

- Depression (very common)
- Dementia
- Psychosis (usually in association with drugs or cortical Lewy body dementia)

Sleep-related manifestations

- Periodic limb movements in sleep and the restless legs syndrome
- REM-sleep behaviour disorder

Dyskinesias

130 Which of the following definitions is correct?

a Dystonia – patterned, sustained involuntary contractions of opposing muscle groups that produce twisting movements or abnormal postures.

b Chorea – rapid, stereotyped, quasi-purposeful involuntary movements.

c Myoclonus – rapid jerky movements that characteristically may be voluntarily suppressed.

d Motor tics – simple, stereotyped, rapid involuntary movements that characteristically cannot be suppressed voluntarily.

e Akathisia – inability to keep still, often waking the patient from sleep at night.

131 With regard to the polymorphic trinucleotide CAG repeat in the gene encoding *Huntingtin*, which of the following statements is true?

a A repeat size ... $(CAG)_{45}$ ... would usually result in Huntington's disease.

b Huntington's disease is transmitted as a Mendelian recessive trait, so two abnormally expanded alleles are necessary to result in a disease phenotype.

c Detection of the expanded trinucleotide repeat is time-consuming and requires gene sequencing.

d A similar repeat sequence in the gene encoding ataxin-1 may be expanded, resulting in dentato-rubro-pallido-luysian atrophy (DRPLA), which is clinically indistinguishable from Huntington's disease.

e The expanded repeat sequence encodes a polylysine region that abolishes the function of the protein.

Each question 132–137 lists an hereditary disease that may be associated with a movement disorder. Match each disease with the protein (from options a to i) that is encoded by the gene bearing the pathogenic mutation for the disease:

a   pantothenate kinase 2

b   hypoxanthine-guanine ribosyl transferase

c   GTP cyclohydrolase 1

d   torsin A

e   atrophin

f ε-sarcoglycan

g   ATPase *ATP7B*

h   glutaryl-CoA-dehydrogenase

i   Kell antigen.

132 Dopa-responsive dystonia.

133 Neuro-acanthocytosis.

134 Wilson's disease.

135 Glutaric aciduria type 1.

136 Hallervorden–Spatz syndrome.

137 Alcohol-responsive myoclonic dystonia.

130

The other definitions should be as follows. Chorea – brief involuntary movements that flow randomly and continuously from one body part to another. Myoclonus – sudden, brief, jerky, shock-like involuntary movements that arise from the CNS and may involve the extremities, face or trunk. Motor tics – brief, co-ordinated, stereotyped involuntary movements that can often be suppressed temporarily, and which are characteristically preceded by a compulsive urge to move that is temporarily relieved by the movement. Akathisia – inability to remain still due to an inner sense of restlessness. This is usually associated with the use of neuroleptic drugs. Although akathisia may make falling asleep difficult, it does not usually cause arousal once the patient is asleep.

131

Huntington's disease is caused by an expanded ... (CAG)$_n$ ... repeat in the gene encoding *Huntingtin*. Repeat sizes of less than 35 have not been associated with disease, and those above 40 are always associated with disease. The CAG sequence encodes glutamine. The resulting protein contains a polyglutamine tract that is expanded in patients with Huntington's disease, giving rise to a

new pathological function that is neurotoxic. The disorder is inherited in an autosomal-dominant pattern; only one copy of the abnormal gene is necessary to produce the disease. DRPLA is more common in Japan than in the UK, is clinically similar to Huntington's disease and is caused by a similar mutation in the gene encoding *Atrophin*.

132

This condition characteristically produces lower limb dystonia with marked diurnal variation and mild parkinsonian signs. Small doses of L-dopa provide dramatic benefit.

133

This condition, which is also called McLeod's syndrome, is associated with orofacial and lingual dystonia, chorea, dementia, an axonal neuropathy and raised serum creatine kinase levels. A clinically similar condition is produced by mutation in a novel gene encoding *Chorein*.

134

The mutation in this Golgi ATPase prevents incorporation of copper into proteins, resulting in loss of caeruloplasmin from the serum and inability to excrete copper in the bile.

135

This is a very rare cause of dystonia in young adults and children.

136

This syndrome is characterised by dystonia, dementia, retinitis pigmentosa and iron deposition in the basal ganglia. Classical childhood-onset Hallervorden–Spatz syndrome is caused by mutations in the *PANK-2* gene; a similar condition in older patients may result from mutations in (i) the *PANK-2* gene, or (ii) the genes encoding caeruloplasmin (acaeruloplasminaemia) or ferritin light chain (neuroferritinopathy), or (iii) other unknown genes.

137

This condition, also known as hereditary essential myoclonus, is characterised by rapid myoclonic jerks, with or without dystonia, which are exquisitely sensitive to alcohol.

Quick fix: Clinical patterns of dystonia

- Generalised – often limbs and trunk; usually childhood onset; often secondary to birth injury or inherited disease.
- Segmental (two adjacent body regions).
- Focal – single site; usually adult onset; commonest sites are neck (torticollis), hand (writer's cramp) and eyelids (blepharospasm).

Quick fix: Causes of dystonia

- Hereditary:
  - primary (idiopathic torsion dystonia, dopa-responsive dystonia, alcohol-responsive myoclonic dystonia)
  - secondary (Huntington's disease; Wilson's disease; Hallervorden–Spatz disease; neuroacanthocytosis; Niemann–Pick disease type C; leukodystrophies; and many more rare diseases).
- Neurodegeneration (Parkinson's disease; multiple system atrophy).
- Drugs (neuroleptics; L-dopa).
- Other acquired disorders (birth asphyxia; kernicterus; basal ganglia tumour; basal ganglia vascular malformation; stroke; cerebral anoxia; cerebral trauma).

Multiple sclerosis I

138 All of the following are commonly encountered sites of clinically manifest lesions in multiple sclerosis *except*:

a medial longitudinal fasciculus

b optic nerve

c cervical spinal cord

d internal segment of globus pallidus

e superior cerebellar peduncle.

139 Which of the following statements best describes the pathology of an acute multiple sclerosis plaque?

a peri-arterial inflammatory changes with pure demyelination

b prominent axonal loss with mild secondary demyelination

c severe perivenous inflammation with axonal destruction

d focal perivenous loss of myelin with relative axonal preservation

e diffuse destruction of large contiguous areas of neuropil, involving neurons and oligodendrocytes.

140 Which of the following statements about an isolated attack of acute retrobulbar neuritis is true?

a   The likelihood of a further clinical event leading to a diagnosis of multiple sclerosis is greater than 95% in the subsequent 5 years.

b   Despite profound visual loss and an afferent papillary defect, the optic disc may appear normal and vision is likely to recover.

c   A diagnosis of multiple sclerosis can be made if the MRI scan shows characteristic abnormalities.

d   The prognosis for visual recovery is improved by early use of corticosteroids.

e   The likelihood of a further clinical event leading to a diagnosis of multiple sclerosis can be greatly reduced by early use of β-interferon.

141 Which of the following statements about the epidemiology of multiple sclerosis is true?

a   The incidence of multiple sclerosis in patients with pernicious anaemia or vitiligo is four times that among the general population.

b   The incidence is much higher at the equator than in Northern Europe

c   The female:male sex ratio is approximately 2.5:1.

d   Few patients have an affected first-degree relative.

e   The concordance rate in monozygotic twins is 95%.

138

Multiple sclerosis (MS) characteristically affects all of the other listed sites (medial longitudinal fasciculus – internuclear ophthalmoplegia; optic nerve – bulbar or retrobulbar neuritis; cervical spine – paraparesis or quadriparesis, which may be asymmetrical and incomplete; cerebellar efferent connection – ataxia and intention tremor). The globus pallidus is not a characteristic site for involvement in MS.

139

The characteristic changes on pathological examination of MS plaques are focal loss of myelin around venules, with relative preservation of axons. This is not the same as pure loss of myelin, and many authors have emphasised that axons are involved in the disease process. Recent work suggests that loss of axons may contribute to the fixed and progressive deficits that are seen in MS.

140

Optic neuritis can give rise to the first symptoms of an illness that subsequently proves clinically to be MS. The probability of this happening is higher if the MRI scan shows white-matter lesions in the brain, but is not affected substantially by the use of β-interferon. Visual recovery is the rule rather than the exception, but steroids do not affect the eventual visual prognosis (although they may help pain associated with optic neuritis, or hasten recovery).

141

The incidence of MS appears to increase away from the equator, although there are exceptions to this (e.g. low incidence in Japan and high incidence in Sardinia). Approximately 15% of patients have an affected relative, and a genetic contribution is suggested by the 25% concordance rate in monozygotic twins compared with the 5% rate in dizygotic twins. The incidence in the context of organ-specific autoimmune diseases is not elevated significantly above background levels.

Quick fix: Diagnosis of multiple sclerosis

- Diagnosis requires the presence of multiple CNS lesions, of the type seen in MS, which satisfy the following conditions:
  - symptoms and signs last for more than 24 hours
  - two or more non-contiguous areas of the CNS are involved ('disseminated in space')
  - two or more lesions occur more than 1 month apart ('disseminated in time')
  - there is no better alternative explanation for the lesions than MS.

- CSF analysis, evoked potential studies and MRI scans are not required to make the diagnosis if the above points can be established clinically.
- If the clinical criteria are not met, dissemination in time may be demonstrated by new enhancing MRI lesions 3 months after a first attack, and dissemination in space may be demonstrated by MRI scanning or evoked potential studies.

Multiple sclerosis II

142 Which of the following statements best describes the role of β-interferon in the treatment of multiple sclerosis?

a β-Interferon reduces the level of clinical disability and the rate of decline in progressive multiple sclerosis.

b β-Interferon reduces the number of relapses that patients have in the first few years after starting treatment.

c β-Interferon reduces the disease burden as seen on MRI scans, with a correlated reduction in fixed disabilities.

d β-Interferon, used after a first attack of demyelination, greatly reduces the proportion of patients who go on to develop clinically definite multiple sclerosis over the subsequent 20 years.

e β-Interferon is free from significant side-effects, but must be given by intravenous infusion to avoid metabolic degradation.

143 With regard to the prognosis for a female patient with a new diagnosis of multiple sclerosis, which of the following statements is true?

a Pregnancy usually precipitates a severe deterioration and should be avoided.

b 50% of patients with relapsing–remitting disease are chair-bound within 5 years of diagnosis.

c An early onset of secondary progression is associated with a worse prognosis.

d Older patients tend to have more slowly progressive disease.

e The prognosis is much improved by the use of β-interferon.

144 Which of the following combinations of findings would allow a clinical diagnosis of multiple sclerosis to be made?

a Optic neuritis; MRI scan shows periventricular white-matter lesions.

b Complete third nerve palsy; MRI shows periventricular white-matter lesions.

c Progressive cerebellar ataxia with raised CSF protein; normal MRI scan.

d Progressive myelopathy with normal brain MRI; CSF shows lymphocytic pleocytosis (300 cells/mL) and oligoclonal IgG bands.

e Spastic paraparesis of new onset; previous history of separate episodes of diplopia and facial anaesthesia that recovered leaving an internuclear ophthalmoplegia; normal MRI.

145 With regard to urinary symptoms in multiple sclerosis, which of the following statements is true?

a The bladder is always spastic.

b The post-void residual volume should be measured to help to determine the mechanism underlying the patient's symptoms.

c Urinary infections are distinctly unusual unless an immunosuppressive drug is being used to treat the multiple sclerosis.

d Intermittent self-catheterisation is inappropriate in the setting of a disease that usually affects vision and upper limb co-ordination.

e An atonic bladder is rarely seen, as this is a lower motor neuron problem and multiple sclerosis is a disease of the CNS.

142

Clinical trials do not show that β-interferon affects the rate of progression of disability, or the prognosis, in progressive multiple sclerosis. The number of relapses is reduced by a third, and the disease burden seen on MRI scanning is also reduced (the dissociation between disability and scan appearance is intriguing). The drug is administered by subcutaneous injection, and therapy can be associated with depression, flu-like symptoms and injection-site reactions.

143

Multiple sclerosis is sufficiently variable that it is impossible to give an accurate prognosis at the onset of the disease. The behaviour of the disease in the early years after diagnosis is the best predictor of prognosis; onset of progression and rapid accumulation of disability predict poor outcome. There is a small increase in relapse rate postpartum, but this is not sufficient for avoidance of pregnancy to be advised. β-Interferon does not affect prognosis unequivocally. Overall, the median time from diagnosis to walking with a stick is 15 years. Older patients tend to have more rapidly progressive disease.

144

Multiple sclerosis is a clinical diagnosis that may be supported by evidence from investigations. Only item **e** describes a multifocal CNS disease in which lesions are disseminated in time and location, without another cause being demonstrated by investigation.

145

Urinary disturbance in multiple sclerosis is complex, and can be related to (i) an atonic bladder that fails to empty completely (usually resulting from a sacral cord lesion or acute spinal shock), (ii) a hyper-reflexic bladder that fails to store urine (resulting from suprasacral CNS disease) or (iii) detrusor-sphincter dyssynergia (resulting from suprasacral spinal disease). As the treatment for each of these is different, it is usually necessary to measure the post-void residual volume by ultrasound or catheter. Urinary infections are very common, especially if there is incomplete emptying. Intermittent self-catheterisation is an effective treatment for an atonic bladder.

Quick fix: Treatment of relapsing–remitting multiple sclerosis

- Pseudorelapses may be triggered by intercurrent illness, which should be treated if appropriate (e.g. urinary infection, pneumonia).
- Corticosteroids do not affect the likelihood or extent of recovery from relapse. They may improve the time course of recovery.
- The frequency of relapses can be reduced by prophylactic use of β-Interferon.
- No treatments unequivocally affect the prognosis with regard to death or disability.

- Symptomatic measures are most important, and include the following:
  - urinary care (treatment of infections, detrusor hyper-reflexia, incomplete emptying)
  - treatment of spasticity
  - treatment of depression
  - care of pressure areas in paraplegic patients.

CNS infections I

146 In the diagnosis of acute bacterial meningitis, which of the following statements is true?

a The CSF is always abnormal.

b A CT brain scan should be undertaken before attempting lumbar puncture.

c CSF analysis is the only way to make a bacteriological diagnosis.

d Antibiotic therapy should be withheld until the CSF sample has been taken.

e Identification of the likely organism is not possible until CSF culture is complete.

147 Which of the following would cast doubt on a diagnosis of viral meningitis?

a reduced conscious level

b CSF lymphocytosis

c headache, nuchal rigidity and fever

d raised CSF protein

e cervical lymphadenopathy.

148 Which of the following organisms is not a common cause of acute bacterial meningitis in adults in the UK?

a   *Neisseria meningitidis*

b   *Borrelia burgdorferi*

c   *Haemophilus influenzae*

d   *Listeria monocytogenes*

e   *Streptococcus pneumoniae.*

149 Which of the following statements about herpes simplex encephalitis is true?

a   A history of recurrent cold sores is required to make the diagnosis.

b   HSV type 2 is usually implicated.

c   Acyclovir has made little difference to the prognosis.

d   Seizures are uncommon.

e   CSF may contain red blood cells and a xanthochromic supernatant.

146

A normal CSF examination excludes the diagnosis. Bacteriological diagnosis can also be made from blood cultures in some cases. CSF microscopy can give helpful clues about the likely pathogen from its morphology and Gram-staining characteristics, and there may also be clinical clues, such as the characteristic rash of meningococcal septicaemia. In the absence of depressed conscious level or focal neurological signs, it is not absolutely necessary to perform a CT scan before undertaking a lumbar puncture, although it is better to do so if in doubt. If there will be a delay before performing the CT/lumbar puncture, it is best to take blood cultures and start high-dose broad-spectrum antibiotic cover immediately, as any delay in treatment may be fatal.

147

Viral meningitis is a benign self-limiting cause of meningism, associated with CSF lymphocytosis, raised protein concentration and (usually) a normal glucose level. Common causes include enteroviruses and the mumps virus, although the cause is not identified in a third of cases. As is usual in systemic viral infections, it is not uncommon to find cervical

lymphadenopathy. The presence of decreased conscious level suggests a diagnosis of encephalitis. Common causes include herpes simplex virus and arboviruses in addition to many of the viruses that can also cause an isolated meningitis, and non-viral causes.

148

Common causes of bacterial meningitis vary with age. In young adults, *Neisseria meningitidis*, *Streptococcus pneumoniae* and *Haemophilus influenzae* (in order of decreasing incidence) account for most cases. In patients over 60 years of age (and pregnant/ immnocompromised patients), *Listeria monocytogenes* is added to the list. *Borrelia burgdorferi* is the causative organism in Lyme disease. It produces an acute lymphocytic meningitis (rather than the classical bacterial picture), and is comparatively rare in the UK.

149

Herpes simplex encephalitis is a serious disease, the prognosis of which has been greatly improved by the availability of acyclovir. Seizures are common, as are confusion, focal signs and fever. Although it is thought to be a reactivation of latent

HSV infection, there is not always a clear history of preceding cold sores. A minority of cases are caused by HSV-2. The severe, haemorrhagic nature of the encephalitis is reflected in the CSF, which may contain red blood cells and their breakdown products, in addition to a lymphocytic pleocytosis and raised protein levels.

Quick fix: CSF in intracranial infections

	Bacterial meningitis	Viral meningitis	TB meningitis	Fungal meningitis
White cell count	↑↑↑ (100–60 000 cells/mm^3, mostly polymorphonuclear cells)	↑↑ (5–500 cells/mm^3, mostly monocytes)	↑↑ (25–500 cells/mm^3, mostly monocytes)	↑↑ (50–800 cells/mm^3, mostly monocytes)
CSF protein	↑↑↑ (1–5 g/l)	Normal or mild ↑ (less than 1 g/l)	↑↑ (1–2 g/l)	↑↑↑ (1–5 g/l)
CSF glucose	↓↓↓ (ratio of CSF: blood glucose <0.3)	Usually normal	↓↓↓ (ratio of CSF: blood glucose <0.3)	↓↓↓ (ratio of CSF: blood glucose <0.3)

Quick fix: CSF white cell and protein levels – correction for traumatic puncture

- Estimation of protein and white cell count can give misleading results if the CSF sample is heavily bloodstained
- The following correction factors may be applied to subtract the components of the white cell count and protein assay that are attributable to bloody contamination:
  - white cell count
    - subtract 1 white cell/mm^3 from total CSF white blood count, for every 700 red blood cells/mm^3
  - CSF protein
    - subtract 0.01 g/l protein from total CSF protein, for every 1000 red blood cells/mm^3
- These correction factors assume that (i) the peripheral full blood count and serum albumin are within normal limits, and (ii) the CSF protein and cell count measurements are carried out on the same sample

CNS infections II

150 Which of the clinical features listed below is compatible with an intracerebral abscess?
(i) Headache worse on coughing and present on waking.
(ii) Generalised tonic–clonic convulsion.
(iii) Right hemiplegia.
(iv) Coma.

a (i) and (iii)

b none of the above

c (i), (ii) and (iii)

d all of the above

e (ii) and (iv).

151 Which of the following statements about the diagnosis of cerebral abscess is true?

a The erythrocyte sedimentation rate (ESR) and C-reactive protein (CRP) are unhelpful as they are often normal.

b The peripheral white blood cell count is usually elevated.

c Fever is almost universal.

d Absence of headache is distinctly unusual.

e Bilateral signs cast doubt on the diagnosis.

152 In neurocysticercosis, which of the following statements is true?

a Affected individuals must have eaten infected pork.

b Epilepsy is unusual; the clinical picture is dominated by meningism.

c The foci of infection are undetectable by MRI, and CSF examination is essential.

d The disease is now uncommon because of an effective vaccination programme in the Third World.

e The role of antihelminthic compounds in treatment is unclear.

153 In meningitis associated with *Mycobacterium tuberculosis*, which of the following statements is true?

a An abnormal chest radiograph is a prerequisite for diagnosis.

b The disease is chronic, and runs its course over a period of weeks.

c Early hydrocephalus is characteristic.

d Mycobacteria are usually visible on the Ziehl–Nielsen (ZN) stain of the CSF.

e Cranial nerve palsy would cast doubt on the diagnosis.

150

Intracerebral abscess can present with effects attributable to raised intracranial pressure, focal deficit or epilepsy. Patients with these clinical presentations should undergo cerebral imaging. Common causes include (i) local spread of infection from the middle ear and mastoid or paranasal air sinuses and (ii) haematogenous spread from bacterial endocarditis or other systemic bacteraemia.

151

Absence of a systemic inflammatory response (with raised inflammatory markers, elevated peripheral white blood cell count and fever) does not exclude the diagnosis of cerebral abscess. It is not unusual for the patient to have little or no headache and to present only with focal deficit or seizures. Bilateral signs may be produced by multiple abscesses or brain displacement leading to false localising signs.

152

Ingestion of eggs, shed per rectum from a human carrying an adult *Taenia solium* tapeworm, may result in (i) infection of a pig, resulting in porcine cysticercosis, or (ii) infection of a human, resulting in human cysticercosis. Both human

autoinfection (5–40% tapeworm carriers) and heteroinfection (contaminated drinking water, infected food handlers) have been described. Thus eating infected pork is not an essential step for acquiring neurocysticercosis. Typical clinical presentations are with seizures, transient focal deficits or raised intracranial pressure. Imaging shows typical changes of cysts in different stages of evolution. There is no effective vaccine, and the disease is a major public health problem in the developing world. The role of anti-helminthic agents remains controversial.

153

TB meningitis can present acutely, does not always occur in individuals with an abnormal chest radiograph, and is associated with basal meningitis causing cranial nerve palsy, and obstruction to the flow of CSF resulting in communicating hydrocephalus. The CSF typically shows lymphocytosis, raised protein and low glucose levels. It is not common to see the mycobacteria in the CSF (< 10% of cases), and culture takes weeks. Polymerase chain reaction (PCR) testing shows sensitivities ranging from 33% to 91%, and specificities ranging from 88% to 100%. The use of the test is still under evaluation.

Quick fix: Causes of recurrent meningitis

Infective causes

- Meningeal disruption (e.g. compound skull fracture with CSF leakage)
- Immunodeficiency states (e.g. complement deficiency, HIV)
- Mollaret's meningitis (herpes simplex virus type 2 infection)

Non-infective causes

- Inflammatory disorders (Behçet's disease, systemic lupus erythematosus, malignant meningitis)
- Drugs (non-steroidal anti-inflammatory drugs, intravenous immunoglobulin, penicillins)
- CNS tumours (epidermoid cysts, craniopharyngiomas, gliomas)

Neurological complications of HIV

154 The differential diagnosis of headache in an HIV-positive patient with a peripheral blood CD4+ lymphocyte count of $350/\mu L$ includes all of the following *except*:

a depression

b cryptococcal meningitis

c migraine

d aseptic meningitis

e zidovudine therapy.

155 All of the following are well-recognised neuromuscular manifestations of primary HIV infection *except*:

a facial nerve palsy

b acute demyelinating polyneuropathy

c brachial neuritis

d cytomegalovirus radiculitis

e acute rhabdomyolysis.

156 Which of the following statements about the AIDS–dementia complex is true?

a   It is not an AIDS-defining illness in the context of chronic HIV infection.

b   Dysphasia and dyspraxia are common findings.

c   Seizures occur in the majority of patients.

d   Loss of fine motor control and action tremor are common findings.

e   The dementia is predominantly cortical, and distributed cognitive processes (e.g. concentration) are rarely affected.

157 In the differential diagnosis of an intracerebral mass lesion in an HIV-positive patient, which of the following favours a diagnosis of *Toxoplasma* brain abscess over primary cerebral lymphoma?

a   a history of co-trimoxazole prophylaxis

b   multiple lesions in cerebral imaging

c   a peripheral blood CD4+ lymphocyte count of 100/μL

d   negative *Toxoplasma* serology

e   persistent low-grade fever.

154

There are many causes of headache in patients with HIV infection, either as a consequence of the disease or of its treatment, or unrelated to either. All of the listed items can cause headaches in patients with HIV, but the CD4+ count is > 200/μL in this patient, effectively excluding opportunistic infections. A chronic, aseptic meningitis is a well-recognised complication of established HIV infection, after the primary infection is established but before the level of immune dysfunction allows opportunistic infections.

155

Primary HIV infection (also called 'seroconversion') may cause a host of systemic symptoms, or may pass without clinical event. The normal CD4 cell count (> 500/μL) on primary infection excludes opportunistic infection with cytomegalovirus (CMV), although a CMV polyradiculopathy can occur in late disease with a CD4 count of < 50/μL.

156

The AIDS–dementia complex is an AIDS-defining illness. It is a subcortical dementia, with prominent slowing of cognition, poor concentration and subtle motor findings. There is usually little to suggest focal cortical dysfunction, and dysphasia and dyspraxia are uncommon. Seizures occur in about 10% of patients. Abnormalities of saccadic eye movement are also common but non-specific. It is important to recognise the condition, as treatment with antiretroviral medications improves the prognosis.

157

The low CD4 count is unhelpful. Both conditions occur in the presence of a CD4 count of < 200/μL – although the median CD4 count is lower in lymphoma, there is much overlap. Co-trimoxazole prophylaxis is very effective in preventing toxoplasmosis. The majority of toxoplasmosis patients have antibodies to *Toxoplasma* resulting from previous infection (these are not present in 10–20% of cases). Persistent fever can occur in either condition. Characteristic imaging findings in toxoplasmosis are multiple enhancing mass lesions, often within the basal ganglia. A single periventricular lesion is more likely to be lymphoma.

Quick fix: Major manifestations of HIV disease in the nervous system

Stage	Blood CD4+ count	Non-focal CNS	Focal CNS	Peripheral nervous system and muscle
Seroconversion	> 500/μL	Headache; meningo-encephalitis	Seizure; myelopathy	Cranial neuropathy; acute polyneuropathy; brachial neuritis; rhabdomyolysis
Moderately advanced	200–500/μL	Chronic meningitis	Tuberculoma	Demyelinating neuropathy; mononeuritis multiplex
AIDS	< 200/μL	AIDS–dementia complex; cryptococcal meningitis; TB meningitis	Toxoplasmosis; primary CNS lymphoma; progressive multifocal leukoencephalopathy; encephalitis (CMV, VZV, HSV)	Painful or sensory polyneuropathy; CMV-related radiculopathy; medication-related and nutritional polyneuropathy

CMV, cytomegalovirus; VZV, varicella zoster virus; HSV, herpes simplex virus.

Brain tumours I

For each of the case scenarios in questions 158–161, choose the most appropriate diagnosis from the list below:

a   low-grade astrocytoma

b   parasagittal meningioma

c   medulloblastoma

d   dysembryoplastic neuroepithelial tumour

e   glioblastoma multiforme.

f   cerebellar haemangioblastoma

g   solitary intracerebral metastasis from lung carcinoma.

158   A 45-year-old man presents with a witnessed generalised convulsion after a late-night party in which he consumed more alcohol than usual. On examination there are no abnormal physical signs. The CT brain scan requested by the Accident and Emergency SHO demonstrates a low-density lesion in the right frontal lobe which shows no pathological enhancement with contrast.

159   A 4-year-old boy presents with gait unsteadiness and falls associated with headache and intermittent vomiting. There is no family history of note. On examination, bilateral optic disc swelling, truncal ataxia and flexor plantar responses are found.

160 A 65-year-old man presents with a 12-month history of intermittent shaking affecting the right leg. The attacks start without warning, commence with jerking in the foot which spreads quickly up the right leg, and last for 1–2 minutes. Afterwards the patient notices a tendency to catch his right foot when he walks for the next 30 minutes. On examination he has mild pyramidal pattern weakness in the right leg and bilateral extensor plantar reflexes.

161 An 18-year-old boy presents with progressive headaches, vomiting and gait disturbance. The headaches are worse in the morning, and the vomiting appears to be associated with rising suddenly from lying down. His brother has recently been seen by an ophthalmologist because of a retinal tumour. On examination there is optic disc swelling and truncal ataxia.

158

Epilepsy is a common presentation of cerebral tumour. Adults who present with a first seizure should undergo neuroimaging. Lesions in the right frontal lobe often produce few if any physical signs. In this case, the site and radiological features most strongly favour a low-grade glioma.

159

Medulloblastoma in particular presents in this age group with progressive cerebellar symptoms and signs. This tumour can spread along the meninges and CSF pathways. The overall prognosis has improved with modern oncological treatment, and the 5-year survival rate is now approximately 70%.

160

Partial motor seizures that commence in the leg suggest a lesion affecting the superior/medial part of the precentral gyrus. Meningiomata often present with seizures, and this diagnosis would be compatible with the long history in this case. The bilateral extensor plantar responses are explained by pressure of the extrinsic tumour on both precentral gyri, which lie adjacent to one another at the vertex. The tumour can obstruct the superior sagittal sinus, causing papilloedema.

161

This patient presents with a progressive cerebellar syndrome and has a family history of retinal tumour. The diagnosis is most likely to be a cerebellar haemangioblastoma secondary to von Hippel–Lindau syndrome. This is an autosomal-dominant syndrome in which haemangioblastomas occur in the CNS and eye. Treatment of the cerebellar lesion is by surgical excision, and screening should be offered to at-risk family members.

Quick fix: Neurocutaneous syndromes

Syndrome	Inheritance	Clinical features
von Hippel–Lindau syndrome	AD	Cerebellar and spinal haemangioblastomata; bilateral renal carcinoma; retinal haemangioblastomata; phaeochromocytoma
Tuberous sclerosis	AD	Shagreen patch; adenoma sebaceum; subungual fibroma; bilateral multiple renal angiomyolipomas; subependymal glial nodules; cortical tuber; cardiac rhabdomyoma
Neurofibromatosis type I	AD	Dermal and plexiform neurofibromata; Lisch nodules; optic nerve glioma; aqueduct stenosis; phaeochromocytoma
Neurofibromatosis type II	AD	Bilateral acoustic neuromata; meningioma; few/no cutaneous signs
Ataxia telangiectasia	AR	Progressive early-onset cerebellar ataxia; ocular telangiectasis large-fibre neuropathy; deficiency of IgA, IgE and IgG2; elevated serum α-fetoprotein, leukaemia and lymphoma

AD, autosomal dominant; AR, autosomal recessive.

Brain tumours II

162 Which of the following statements about acoustic neuroma is *incorrect*?

a It can be associated with elevated CSF protein levels.

b Bilateral tumours are frequently seen in neurofibromatosis type I.

c It commonly causes painless unilateral hearing loss.

d It may present with hydrocephalus.

e Papilloedema is a recognised physical sign.

163 Which of the following intracerebral tumours is *not* commonly associated with calcification on CT brain scan?

a glioblastoma multiforme

b ependymoma

c craniopharyngioma

d oligodendroglioma

e central neurocytoma.

164 Which of the following statements about the presentation of primary brain tumours is *incorrect*?

a They frequently present with chronic daily headaches in isolation.

b They may present with focal limb weakness without papilloedema.

c They can be associated with generalised seizures without clear partial onset.

d They occasionally cause paroxysmal symptoms reminiscent of transient ischaemic attacks.

e They are often associated with personality change or depression.

165 Which of the following primary tumours is *least* likely to be associated with intracerebral metastasis?

a malignant melanoma

b squamous-cell lung carcinoma

c breast carcinoma

d colon carcinoma

e prostate carcinoma.

162

Acoustic neuroma usually presents with painless unilateral sensorineural hearing loss, sometimes associated with tinnitus and vertigo. MRI of the internal auditory meatus is a sensitive way to identify the tumour, which may be associated with obstructive hydrocephalus if the fourth ventricle is compressed. An elevated CSF protein concentration is common. Bilateral acoustic neuromata are a feature of neurofibromatosis type II.

163 (a)

Many types of chronic cerebral pathology are frequently associated with calcification (see *Quick fix* opposite). The highly malignant glioblastoma multiforme does not characteristically calcify.

164

Brain tumours rarely present with chronic daily headache in isolation, focal neurological deficit or epilepsy being much more common. Headache from raised intracranial pressure is typically present on waking, eased by standing and associated with early-morning nausea and vomiting, papilloedema and visual obscurations.

165

Prostate carcinoma tends to metastasise to bone. In the head, this typically results in skull metastasis rather than an intraparenchymal cerebral lesion. Common tumours that metastasise to the brain parenchyma include those of the lung, breast and colon, and melanoma.

Quick fix: Clinical presentation of intracranial space-occupying lesion

Focal neurological deficit

- Hemiparesis/hemisensory (43%)
- Cognitive/personality (27%)
- Dysphasia (14%)
- Hemianopia (10%)

Epileptic seizure(s)

Raised intracranial pressure

- Headache
- Papilloedema (14%)
- Bradycardia
- Nausea/vomiting
- Abducens (VI) nerve palsy ('false localising')

Endocrine (rare)

- Diabetes insipidus
- Syndrome of inappropriate antidiuretic hormone secretion (SIADH)
- Hyperprolactinaemia

Quick fix: Causes of intracranial calcification

- Physiological – pineal; choroids; falx; tentorium
- Developmental – tuberose sclerosis; Sturge–Weber syndrome
- Tumour – craniopharyngioma (90%); oligodendroglioma (90%); central neurocytoma (70%); ependymoma (50%); meningioma (25%)
- Infection – congenital (toxoplasmosis, cytomegalovirus, rubella, herpes simplex); parasite (neurocysticercosis, echinococcus); tuberculosis; syphilis; fungal (histoplasmosis, coccidioidomycosis)
- Metabolic – hypoparathyroidism; hypercalcaemia; pseudohypoparathyroidism; lead; hypothyroidism; mitochondrial disease
- Vascular – aneurysm; arteriovenous malformation

Disorders of intracranial pressure

For each of the case scenarios in questions 166–169, choose the most appropriate diagnosis from the list below:

a spontaneous intracranial hypotension

b cerebral venous sinus thrombosis

c idiopathic intracranial hypertension

d normal-pressure hydrocephalus

e obstructive hydrocephalus

f communicating hydrocephalus.

166 A 24-year-old female patient presents with a history of 2 months of increasing headache and episodes of 'greying out' of vision in the right eye. These typically occur in the morning and last for 30–60 seconds. She is overweight, and has recently gained a further 10 kg after giving up aerobics due to time pressures. Fundoscopy discloses optic disc swelling, which is worse in the right eye, where haemorrhages are visible around the disc.

167 A 19-year-old female patient presents with headache, drowsiness and episodes of left leg and arm shaking, all of which have evolved rapidly over a few days. She has recently started the combined oral contraceptive pill. Examination reveals mild optic disc swelling and a left extensor plantar response.

168 A 24-year-old man returns from a visit to Jamaica complaining of drowsiness, headaches and unsteadiness. He recalls developing a severe sudden-onset headache 2 weeks previously, which was associated with neck stiffness, nausea and vomiting. He did not seek medical attention at the time, and the symptoms started to resolve after 5 days, until he became drowsy and unsteady 4 days ago. Examination reveals mild nuchal rigidity and extensor plantar responses.

169 A 65-year-old man complains of severe headaches, which started abruptly 2 days ago following an upper respiratory tract viral infection with pronounced violent coughing. The headache, which is associated with nausea and tinnitus, occurs soon after rising in the morning and is abolished by lying flat in bed. There are no abnormal focal neurological findings.

166

The majority of patients with idiopathic intracranial hypertension are female with a high body mass index and a history of recent weight gain. Headaches and papilloedema (with visual obscuration) are typical. Nausea and vomiting are rare, as is sixth nerve palsy. Importantly, there are no focal signs. The diagnosis is confirmed by a normal MRI brain scan and a lumbar puncture demonstrating an elevated opening pressure with normal CSF constituents.

167

Cerebral venous sinus thrombosis presents with raised intracranial pressure, focal neurological deficit and seizures. The differential diagnosis includes viral encephalitis and intracranial mass lesion. Thrombi in the venous sinuses may be visible on MRI.

168

This patient suffered a subarachnoid haemorrhage while abroad, and now presents with hydrocephalus. This is likely to be communicating, because the presence of blood in the subarachnoid space impairs the absorption of CSF by the arachnoid granulations. Appropriate management would include a CT brain scan followed by lumbar puncture or a temporary shunt and referral for four-vessel cerebral angiography.

169

Spontaneous intracranial hypotension usually presents with orthostatic headache similar to that which occurs after lumbar puncture. CSF leakage from the spinal subarachnoid space can occasionally be demonstrated. Management is symptomatic, as most cases resolve spontaneously. In intractable cases, a spinal blood patch may be helpful.

Quick fix: Causes of raised intracranial pressure

Mass lesion

- Tumour
- Haematoma (subdural, extradural, intraparenchymal)
- Abscess
- Granuloma

Oedema

- Head injury
- Hypoxia
- Metabolic/toxic causes (liver failure, urea cycle defects, lead poisoning)

Intracranial inflammation

- Encephalitis
- Meningitis
- Acute demyelinating encephalomyelitis

Vascular disease

- Cerebral venous sinus thrombosis
- Cerebral infarction

Miscellaneous

- Idiopathic intracranial hypertension
- Communicating and obstructive hydrocephalus
- Hypertensive encephalopathy

Migraine and benign headaches

170 Which of the following statements about migraine is *incorrect?*

a It affects females more frequently than males.

b It may cause EEG abnormalities.

c It can rarely be associated with a unilateral fixed dilated pupil.

d Diagnosis is unlikely if nuchal rigidity and fever are present in an acute attack.

e An MRI brain scan should be performed to confirm the diagnosis.

171 With mutations in which of the following genes (which encode neuronal ion channels) is familial hemiplegic migraine associated?

a *CHRNA4* – nicotinic acetylcholine receptor

b *KCNQ2* – voltage-gated potassium channel

c *CLCN1* – voltage-gated chloride channel

d *CACNL1A* – voltage-gated calcium channel

e *SCN4A* – voltage-gated sodium channel.

172 Which acute treatment would be most suitable for a 55-year-old woman with twice-monthly migrainous headaches associated with vomiting but no aura, and a history of chronic stable exertional angina on low-dose (75 mg) aspirin?

a   propranolol

b   subcutaneous sumatriptan

c   tolfenamic acid (200 mg) and metoclopramide (10 mg)

d   pizotifen

e   ergotamine.

173 Which of the following is not a typical feature of acute cluster headaches?

a   severe headache lasting 24 hours

b   rhinorrhoea

c   unilateral ptosis

d   significant relief of symptoms with high-flow oxygen

e   lacrimation.

170

Migraine is more common in females than in males, and may be associated with EEG abnormalities. A fixed dilated pupil without external ophthalmoplegia may rarely be seen after an attack. Hemiplegic migraine is uncommon and often familial (however, a hemisensory aura is common). An MRI brain scan is useful for excluding other disorders, but is of no use in confirming the diagnosis, which is clinical.

171

Familial hemiplegic migraine is associated with mutations in the gene encoding the α_{1A} subunit of the neuronal voltage-gated calcium channel (*CACNL1A*). Patients present with migrainous headaches associated with hemiparesis, often with drowsiness or fever. The differential diagnosis at first presentation includes viral encephalitis and cerebral venous sinus thrombosis.

172

Propranolol and pizotifen are useful in the prophylaxis of migraine, but are of little value during an acute attack. Both ergotamine and sumatriptan are contraindicated if there is significant coronary artery disease. Non-steroidal anti-inflammatory drugs, such as tolfenamic acid or high-dose aspirin, together with metoclopramide are efficacious in the acute treatment of migraine.

173

Cluster headaches typically affect middle-aged male smokers, and are part of a spectrum of benign headaches called trigeminal autonomic cephalalgias. The attacks last for less than 180 minutes. The other listed features are all typical.

Quick fix: Trigeminal autonomic cephalalgias

	Cluster headache	Paroxysmal hemicrania	SUNCT
Typical site of pain	Periorbital	Periorbital/frontal	Unilateral headache
Autonomic features	Ipsilateral rhinorrhoea, lacrimation, sweating, nasal obstruction, eyelid swelling, ptosis, Horner's syndrome, red eye, asymmetrical flushing or sweating	Ipsilateral lacrimation, rhinorrhoea and conjunctival injection	Ipsilateral conjunctival injection and lacrimation ('tearing')
Duration of attack	30–180 minutes	5–20 minutes	30 seconds to 2 minutes
Frequency of attacks	1–3 attacks/day	5–20 attacks/day	10 attacks/hour
Treatment	Acute: subcutaneous sumatriptan; 100% O_2 Prophylaxis: verapamil; prednisolone	Indomethacin (response to indomethacin is required to make the diagnosis)	Anticonvulsants (lamotrigine; gabapentin; topiramate)

SUNCT, **s**hort-lasting **u**nilateral **n**euralgiform headache with **c**onjunctival injection and **t**earing.

Spinal cord diseases

174 In which of the following disorders are absent knee reflexes and extensor plantar responses characteristically seen?

a thoracic spine meningioma

b extradural spinal cord compression

c multiple sclerosis

d cervical spondylitic myelopathy

e subacute combined degeneration of the spinal cord secondary to vitamin B$_{12}$ deficiency.

175 A 43-year-old Jamaican woman presents with a 5-year history of slowly progressive gait instability and impaired bladder function. Examination reveals a spastic paraparesis, without sensory abnormality. An MRI scan of the spinal cord is normal. The CSF shows 2 lymphocytes with a CSF protein concentration of 0.6 g/L. The venereal disease research laboratory test (VDRL) is positive in blood but negative in CSF. What is the most likely diagnosis?

a neurosarcoidosis

b TB meningitis

c Lyme disease

d human T lymphotropic virus type 1 (HTLV-1) associated myelopathy

e neurosyphilis.

176 A 65-year-old man with hypertension presents with a 1-year history of progressive back pain, stiffness and weakness in the legs and urinary incontinence. Examination reveals a spastic paraparesis with a sensory level at T9. There is no clinical evidence of aortic disease, and no spinal bruits can be heard. The MRI scan shows marked swelling of the low thoracic cord together with prominent flow voids and a serpiginous lesion on gradient echo sequences. What is the most likely diagnosis?

a spinal dural arteriovenous (AV) fistula

b spontaneous haematomyelia

c thoracic cord astrocytoma

d anterior spinal artery thrombosis

e multiple sclerosis.

177 Which of the following is *not* a recognised cause of myelitis?

a varicella zoster

b *Borrelia burgdorferi*

c schistosomiasis

d leprosy

e Japanese B encephalitis.

174

Absent knee reflexes and extensor plantars may be seen in Friedreich's ataxia, syphilitic taboparesis, motor neuron disease, conus medullaris lesions and subacute combined degeneration of the spinal cord.

175

HTLV-1 associated myelopathy typically presents with a slowly progressive spinal cord syndrome in patients from the West Indies or parts of Japan. Inflammatory myositis, peripheral neuropathy and vestibulocochlear (VIII) cranial nerve involvement are rare additional features. Diagnosis rests on the demonstration of antibodies to HTLV-1 in blood and CSF with normal spinal imaging.

176

This patient presents with a slowly progressive myelopathy, making anterior spinal artery thrombosis and haematomyelia (spinal cord haemorrhage) unlikely. The MRI scan demonstrates a serpiginous lesion with flow voids, which is the typical appearance of a spinal dural arteriovenous fistula. Spinal angiography is required to confirm the diagnosis, and treatment is by either embolisation or surgical ligation of the fistula.

177

Lyme disease (*Borrelia burgdorferi*), varicella zoster, syphilis and schistosomiasis are all well-recognised causes of myelitis. Japanese B encephalitis has recently been recognised as causing a poliomyelitis-like illness with flaccid tetraplegia. Leprosy causes a peripheral neuritis as opposed to myelitis.

Quick fix: Causes of spinal cord disease

- Inherited disorders (hereditary spastic paraparesis, Friedreich's ataxia, adrenomyeloneuropathy)
- Developmental disorders (neural-tube defect)
- Mass lesion:
  - extradural compression (metastatic disease, spondylosis, epidural abscess)
  - intradural extramedullary compression (meningioma, neurofibroma)
  - intradural intramedullary lesion (astrocytoma, ependymoma, syringomyelia, haematomyelia)
- Inflammation:
  - multiple sclerosis
  - isolated acute transverse myelitis
  - neurosarcoidosis
  - Devic's disease (neuromyelitis optica)
- Infection:
  - viral (HIV, HTLV-1, herpes viruses)
  - bacterial (syphilis, brucellosis, borreliosis)
  - parasitic (schistosomiasis)
- Vascular causes:
  - anterior spinal artery occlusion
  - dural arteriovenous fistula
- Metabolic causes:
  - vitamin B_{12} deficiency

Motor neuron disease

178 Familial amyotrophic lateral sclerosis has been associated with mutations in the gene encoding:

a aryl sulphatase A

b glucosidase

c β-galactosidase

d superoxide dismutase

e sphingomyelinase.

179 Which of the following would exclude a diagnosis of motor neuron disease (MND)?

a lymphocytic CSF with raised CSF protein level

b delayed central motor conduction time

c mildly elevated serum creatine kinase level

d sensory symptoms

e flexor plantar responses.

180 A 64-year-old man has lost the function in his hands over a period of 3 months and now complains of difficulty in walking. Examination reveals bilateral wasting of the thenar and hypothenar eminences, which is worse on the right, where the biceps reflex is absent. There is a mild spastic paraparesis with a few fasciculations in the left quadriceps. Which of the following statements is correct?

a A myelopathy is excluded by the presence of lower motor neuron signs.

b A test for antibodies to acetylcholine receptors (anti-AChR) should be requested.

c The absence of denervation in the lower limbs on electromyogram (EMG) examination would exclude the diagnosis of motor neuron disease.

d A CSF examination is likely to be helpful, as it would demonstrate the characteristic changes of motor neuron disease.

e An MRI scan of the cervical spine is essential for excluding a structural lesion.

181 Which of the following statements about motor neuron disease is correct?

a The incidence of motor neuron disease is highest in the fifth decade.

b Riluzole has proven efficacy in the management of patients with the progressive muscular atrophy variant of motor neuron disease.

c The prognosis is adversely affected by the development of bulbar symptoms.

d The proportion of familial cases is around 30%.

e Involvement of the extra-ocular muscles is frequently seen early in the disease.

178

Familial motor neuron disease is uncommon; 20% of familial cases are associated with mutations in the gene encoding superoxide dismutase (SOD-1, autosomal dominant). The remaining enzymes are associated with the following: aryl sulphatase A – metochromatic leucodystrophy; glucosidase – Gaucher's disease; β-galactosidase – GM1 gangliosidosis; sphingomyelinase – Niemann–Pick's disease types A and B.

179

Sensory symptoms (but not signs) are frequently found in motor neuron disease. Serum creatine kinase levels may be raised if there is rapid widespread denervation. An inflammatory CSF with lymphocytosis and elevated protein levels effectively excludes the diagnosis, and should raise the possibility of other conditions, such as malignant meningitis, Lyme disease, syphilis and neurosarcoidosis.

180

This patient has lower motor neuron signs in the arms and upper motor neuron signs in the legs, raising the possibility of a focal lesion in the cervical spine, which should be imaged. This is unlikely to be a presentation of myasthenia gravis. There are no typical CSF changes in motor neuron disease, and a lumbar puncture should be performed only to exclude other disorders.

181

The incidence of motor neuron disease rises with age and peaks in the eighth decade. Riluzole has a modest disease-modifying action in the amyotrophic lateral sclerosis form of motor neuron disase. Bulbar symptoms and signs in motor neuron disease are associated with a poor prognosis. The extra-ocular muscles are never affected early in the disease, but may be a feature in end-stage patients who have been maintained on mechanical ventilation for prolonged periods.

Quick fix: Diseases that can mimic motor neuron disease

- Structural disease of the brainstem and spinal cord
- Pure lower motor neuron syndromes:
  - multifocal motor neuropathy with conduction block
  - spinal muscular atrophy
  - X-linked spinal and bulbar muscular atrophy
  - benign focal amyotrophy (Hiroyama's disease)
  - hexosaminidase A deficiency (adult-onset Tay–Sachs disease)

- Neuromuscular junction disorder:
  - myasthenia gravis
- Myopathies:
  - inclusion body myositis

Dementia

182 Each of the following is a well-recognised clinical feature of Alzheimer's disease *except*:

a myoclonus

b widespread muscle fasciculations

c apraxia

d generalised seizures

e dyscalculia.

183 Which of the following factors is epidemiologically associated with a reduced incidence of Alzheimer's disease?

a increased age

b head injury

c cigarette smoking

d prolonged use of non-steroidal anti-inflammatory drugs (NSAIDs)

e apolipoprotein $\varepsilon 4$ genotype.

184 Which of the following statements about variant Creutzfeldt–Jakob disease (CJD) is *incorrect*?

a Early sensory symptoms are a recognised feature.

b 14-3-3 protein is detected in the CSF more frequently than in sporadic CJD.

c MRI brain scans may show high-signal lesions bilaterally in the pulvinar nucleus of the thalamus on T2-weighted and FLAIR sequences.

d Affected patients may present to psychiatrists with depression.

e All patients to date have been homozygous for methionine at the polymorphic position 129 of the prion protein gene.

185 Which of the following neuropathological findings is *not* a characteristic feature of Alzheimer's disease?

a neuritic plaques

b amyloid angiopathy

c subcortical infarcts

d neuronal loss

e neurofibrillary tangles.

182

Myoclonus and seizures are rare but well-described features of Alzheimer's disease. Widespread fasciculations are more commonly associated with variants of frontotemporal dementia.

183

Recognised risk factors for Alzheimer's disease include increased age and the apolipoprotein $\varepsilon 4$ genotype. There are conflicting data on the role of head injury (probably increased risk) and smoking (probably no effect), but neither factor has been shown to be protective. However, there is increasing evidence that prolonged use of NSAIDs (> 2 years) is associated with a reduced incidence of Alzheimer's disease.

184

New variant CJD (vCJD) is believed to be associated with bovine spongiform encephalopathy, and may present in the early stages with psychiatric features and sensory symptoms. MRI brain scans may show high-signal lesions in the pulvinar nucleus of the thalamus on FLAIR and T2-weighted images. However, 14-3-3 protein is less often positive in CSF compared with sporadic CJD, and the EEG may not show the characteristic triphasic potentials. All of the individuals affected to date have been homozygous for methionine at position 129 of the prion protein gene.

185

Lacunar infarcts and ischaemic white-matter lesions associated with small-vessel disease are commonly associated with vascular dementia, and may coexist with Alzheimer's disease, but are not part of the characteristic neuropathological picture.

Quick fix: Treatable causes of dementia

- Tumour:
  - olfactory groove meningioma
  - benign tumour of third ventricle
- Infection:
  - syphilis
  - HIV
  - Whipple's disease
  - Lyme disease
- Inflammatory causes:
  - Hashimoto's encephalopathy
  - limbic encephalitis

- Metabolic disorders:
  - hypothyroidism
  - vitamin B_{12} deficiency
  - liver and renal failure
- Miscellaneous causes:
  - hydrocephalus
  - cerebral vasculitis
  - systemic lupus erythematosus-associated micro-angiopathy

Peripheral neuropathy I

186 With which of the following inherited peripheral neuropathies are duplications in the *PMP22* gene associated?

a Charcot–Marie–Tooth disease type 1a

b hereditary liability to pressure palsies

c Charcot–Marie–Tooth disease type 2

d giant axonal neuropathy

e Refsum's disease.

187 Which of the following signs is *not* characteristically associated with acute Guillain–Barré syndrome?

a areflexia

b flexor plantar responses

c impaired proprioception

d bilateral facial paralysis

e pinprick sensory level on the trunk.

188 Which of the following statements about intravenous immunoglobulin is *incorrect?*

a Adverse effects include aseptic meningitis.

b It is inferior to plasma exchange in the management of Guillain–Barré syndrome.

c It is associated with improved speed of recovery in Guillain–Barré syndrome.

d It is contraindicated in patients with selective IgA deficiency.

e It is the treatment of choice for multifocal motor neuropathy with conduction block.

189 The characteristic features of the POEMS syndrome include all of the following *except*:

a papilloedema

b mixed axonal and demyelinating neuropathy

c low testosterone levels in males

d small-cell lung carcinoma

e hepatomegaly.

186

Hereditary motor and sensory neuropathies (HMSN) (Charcot–Marie–Tooth disease) can be divided into demyelinating (type 1) and axonal (type 2) forms. HMSN type 1a is associated with a duplication in the *PMP22* gene. Deletions in the same gene give rise to hereditary neuropathy with liability to pressure palsies. HMSN type 2 is associated with axonal pathology, and mutations have been described in genes encoding neurofilament light chain, kinesin motor protein 1b and myelin protein zero gene.

187

A sensory level on the trunk is not a feature of Guillain–Barré syndrome, and a spinal cord lesion should be sought.

188

Intravenous immunoglobulin has been demonstrated to be effective in a range of immunologically mediated neurological conditions, including Guillain–Barré syndrome, chronic inflammatory demyelinating polyneuropathy and myasthenia gravis. It is contraindicated in patients with selective IgA deficiency. The efficacy of intravenous immunoglobulin in Guillain–Barré syndrome is equal to that of plasma exchange.

189

The POEMS syndrome is a rare paraproteinaemic neuropathy that is found in association with an osteosclerotic myeloma. It is characterised by **p**olyneuropathy (typically mixed axonal and demyelinating), **o**rganomegaly, **e**ndocrinopathy (abnormal thyroid function and low testosterone levels), **m**onoclonal gammopathy and **s**kin changes. Papilloedema is found in a proportion of cases. There is no association with small-cell lung cancer.

Quick fix: Causes of chronic demyelinating peripheral neuropathy

- Inherited causes:
  - hereditary motor and sensory neuropathy (HMSN) types 1 and 3
  - hereditary neuropathy with liability to pressure palsy
  - adrenoleucodystrophy
  - Refsum's disease
- Acquired causes:
  - chronic inflammatory demyelinating polyneuropathy (CIDP)
  - multifocal motor neuropathy (MMN) with conduction block
  - paraproteinaemic neuropathies
- Toxic causes
  - amiodarone
  - perhexiline

Quick fix: Causes of motor peripheral neuropathy

- Hereditary motor and sensory neuropathy
- Porphyria
- Guillain–Barré syndrome
- Acute motor axonal neuropathy
- Multifocal motor neuropathy with conduction block
- Diphtheria
- Toxic (dapsone, lead, organophosphates)

Quick fix: Causes of sensory–ataxic peripheral neuropathy

- Deficiency (vitamins B_{12} and E)
- Diabetes mellitus
- Sjögren's syndrome
- Paraneoplastic sensory neuropathy
- Hereditary sensory and autonomic neuropathy
- CANOMAD (**c**hronic **a**taxic **n**europathy with **o**phthalmoplegia, **M**-protein, cold **a**gglutinins and **d**isialosyl antibodies)

Peripheral neuropathy II

190 All of the following drugs are associated with an axonal peripheral neuropathy *except*:

a simvastatin

b isoniazid

c stavudine

d tacrolimus

e phenytoin.

191 A 23-year-old male patient presents with paraesthesia in his feet, followed by rapidly evolving ascending weakness, having recently returned from a 3-month business trip to the Far East. On examination he has mild facial weakness and severe flaccid symmetrical quadraparesis with areflexia. Nerve conduction studies show evidence of a demyelinating polyneuropathy. CSF studies reveal 168 lymphocytes/mL, and a protein concentration of 1.8 g/L. Which of the following statements is correct?

a A diagnosis of Guillain–Barré syndrome may be made with confidence.

b An MRI scan of the brain and spine is essential.

c Treatment with aciclovir is indicated.

d Intravenous immunoglobulin therapy is inappropriate.

e Informed consent for an HIV test should be obtained.

192 Which of the following autoantibodies is particularly associated with the Miller–Fisher variant of Guillain–Barré syndrome (ophthalmoplegia, ataxia and areflexia)?

a   anti-GQ1b antibodies

b   anti-GM1 antibodies

c   anti-calcium-channel antibodies

d   anti-potassium-channel antibodies

e   anti-neuronal antibodies.

193 A 45-year-old woman presents with a 2-week history of pain and weakness initially commencing in her right foot and then spreading to affect her left hand. There is a past history of severe asthma requiring systemic steroid treatment, but the steroid dose has been reduced in the last 6 months with the introduction of a leukotriene antagonist, montelukast.
On examination there is evidence of right common peroneal nerve, left anterior interosseous nerve and left median nerve palsies. Routine blood tests show an erythrocyte sedimentation rate of 65 mm/hour and an eosinophil count of 4×10^9/mL. What is the most likely diagnosis?

a   malignant meningitis

b   sarcoidosis

c   Churg–Strauss syndrome

d   polyarteritis nodosa

e   mixed essential cryoglobulinaemia.

190

All of the drugs listed are associated with an axonal neuropathy except for tacrolimus, which is associated with a demyelinating neuropathy.

191 (e)

Guillain–Barré syndrome is excluded in this patient because of the high CSF lymphocyte count. The most likely diagnosis is primary HIV infection ('seroconversion illness') presenting with an acute demyelinating polyneuropathy. Intravenous immunoglobulin treatment is not contraindicated in HIV disease.

192

Miller–Fisher syndrome is associated with antibodies to the ganglioside GQ1b. Antibodies to another ganglioside (GM1) have been found in Guillain–Barré syndrome (particularly in association with preceding *Campylobacter* infection), as well as in multifocal motor neuropathy with conduction block. A chronic sensory ataxic neuropathy known as CANOMAD (**c**hronic **a**taxic **n**europathy with **o**phthalmoplegia, **M**-protein, cold **a**gglutinins and **d**isialosyl antibodies) has recently been described in association with high titres of anti-GQ1b antibody.

193

Churg–Strauss syndrome is suggested by the 'mononeuritis multiplex' pattern of the neuropathy, the history of severe asthma and the raised eosinophil count. It is recognised that patients may present after starting treatment with a leukotriene antagonist, although this may be due to the unmasking of underlying disease with corticosteroid withdrawal.

Quick fix: Causes of death in acute Guillain–Barré syndrome

- Deep vein thrombosis (DVT), thrombo-embolism (limb paralysis)
- Respiratory failure (respiratory muscle weakness)
- Pneumonia/aspiration (bulbar and respiratory muscle weakness)
- Cardiac arrhythmia (autonomic involvement)

Quick fix: Management of acute Guillain–Barré syndrome

Supportive measures

- Airway – may require endotracheal intubation if unable to protect airway
- Prophylaxis against deep venous thrombosis
- Nutrition – may require nasogastric tube if there is bulbar dysfunction
- Analgesia for back and limb pain
- Care of pressure areas, bladder and bowels if patient is immobile

Monitoring

- Respiratory monitoring:
  - regular measurement of slow vital capacity (SVC)
  - ITU referral if SVC is less than 15 ml/kg (i.e. 1 L for a 65 kg adult); may require ventilation
- Cardiac monitoring:
  - ECG monitoring
  - cardiological advice if there is haemodynamically significant or sustained arrhythmia; may require temporary pacing wire or drugs

Immunomodulatory treatment

- Intravenous immunoglobulin (0.4 g/kg/day for 5 days)
  or
- Plasma exchange

Neuromuscular junction disorders

194 Which of the following statements about the investigation of myasthenia gravis is *incorrect*?

a A negative anti-AChR antibody titre does not exclude the diagnosis.

b Single-fibre electromyography (EMG) is a sensitive but not specific test for myasthenia gravis.

c A positive Tensilon test is not required to confirm the diagnosis.

d False positive anti-AChR titres are extremely rare.

e A normal chest radiograph is sufficient to exclude thymoma.

195 Which of the following features is most useful for distinguishing myasthenia gravis from the Lambert–Eaton myasthenic syndrome?

a ptosis

b proximal muscle weakness with fatiguability

c abnormal single-fibre EMG

d symptoms of autonomic dysfunction

e negative anti-AChR antibodies.

196 A 72-year-old woman presents with a 1-month history of increasing dysarthria and dysphagia together with fatiguable ptosis and diplopia. Her anti-AChR titre is strongly positive. Which of the following statements is correct?

a Intravenous immunoglobulin therapy is unlikely to prove effective.

b Single-fibre EMG is not required to confirm the diagnosis.

c Azathioprine therapy would be expected to cause rapid symptom improvement.

d Steroids should be started at 1.5 mg/kg/day together with treatment to prevent osteoporosis.

e An MRI brain scan is essential.

197 Which of the following drugs is *least* likely to exacerbate weakness in a patient with myasthenia gravis?

a gentamicin

b erythromycin

c ciprofloxacin

d telithromycin

e ceftriaxone.

194

Around 10–15% of patients with generalised myasthenia gravis and 50% of patients with purely ocular myasthenia gravis do not have detectable antibodies to acetylcholine receptors. Recently, antibodies to muscle-specific kinase (MuSK) have been detected in around 40% of patients with seronegative generalised (but not ocular) myasthenia gravis. A negative chest X-ray does not exclude thymoma, and a CT scan of the thorax should be requested.

195

In Lambert–Eaton myasthenic syndrome (LEMS), autoantibodies are directed against presynaptic P/Q-type voltage-gated calcium channels. Fatiguable muscle weakness occurs in a similar distribution to myasthenia gravis, although the extra-ocular muscles and diaphragm are much less frequently affected in LEMS. Autonomic symptoms are common in LEMS but typically absent in myasthenia gravis.

196

These are characteristic features of generalised myasthenia gravis, and single-fibre EMG is not required to make the diagnosis. Treatment with intravenous immunoglobulin is likely to improve symptoms rapidly over 7–14 days. Prednisolone should be started, but at a low dose in order to avoid precipitating a myasthenic crisis. Azathioprine may be used for a steroid-sparing effect, but it may take 12–18 months for this to occur.

197

Drugs that impair neuromuscular transmission include several different classes of antibiotics (macrolides, quinolones and aminoglycosides), as well as depolarising and non-depolarising muscle relaxants (e.g. pancuronium) and calcium-channel blockers.

Quick fix: Disorders of the neuromuscular junction

	Myasthenia gravis	LEMS	Botulism
Muscles typically affected	Extra-ocular, bulbar, facial, axial, respiratory with or without proximal limb muscles	Axial and proximal limb muscles	Early: extra-ocular and facial muscles Late: generalised limb and bulbar weakness
Autonomic features	None	Dry mouth, impotence, constipation	Mydriasis, dry mouth
Associated tumour	Thymoma	Small-cell lung carcinoma	None
Cause	Autoantibodies against postsynaptic acetylcholine receptor or MuSK	Autoantibodies against presynaptic voltage-gated calcium channel	Exotoxin secreted by *Clostridium botulinum* disrupts function of presynaptic terminal
Neurophysiology	Abnormal single-fibre EMG; CMAP decreases on repetitive stimulation	Abnormal single-fibre EMG; small CMAP amplitude is markedly increased after voluntary contraction	Abnormal single-fibre EMG

LEMS, Lambert–Eaton myasthenic syndrome; MuSK, muscle-specific kinase; CMAP, compound muscle action potential.

Muscle disease

198 Which of the following is *not* a recognised feature of facioscapulohumeral (FSH) dystrophy linked to chromosome 4q?

a   tibialis anterior weakness

b   unilateral winging of the scapula

c   cataract

d   relative preservation of the deltoid muscle

e   exudative retinal detachment.

199 Which of the following statements about dermatomyositis is *incorrect*?

a   It shares an identical muscle histopathology with polymyositis.

b   A normal creatine phosphokinase (CPK) level does not exclude the diagnosis.

c   Concentric needle EMG may reveal small-amplitude short-duration muscle action potentials with positive sharp waves and fibrillations.

d   It responds to treatment with prednisolone.

e   In older adults, it may be associated with an underlying internal malignancy.

200 Which of the following muscular dystrophies is *not* associated with cardiac involvement?

a   Emery–Dreifuss muscular dystrophy

b   myotonic dystrophy

c   Becker muscular dystrophy

d   oculopharyngeal muscular dystrophy

e   Duchenne muscular dystrophy.

201 Which of the following conditions is *not* commonly associated with muscle disease?

a   hypothyroidism

b   hyperglycaemia

c   hyperparathyroidism

d   hyperthyroidism

e   Cushing's syndrome.

198

FSH dystrophy shows autosomal-dominant inheritance. There is > 90% penetrance by 20 years of age, but a few cases present in the third and fourth decades. The muscle weakness is slowly progressive. Recognised extramuscular features include deafness and exudative retinal detachment, but not cataract.

199

Dermatomyositis presents classically with a heliotrope skin rash (periorbital, chest, hands) and predominantly proximal muscle weakness. There may also be malaise and weight loss. Pathologically, there is vasculitis affecting the blood vessels in muscle, giving rise to ischaemic damage. In contrast, polymyositis is associated with an inflammatory lymphocytic infiltrate into muscle with no evidence of vasculitis. Both conditions may be associated with underlying malignancy in older patients.

200

Cardiac involvement is an important cause of morbidity in Duchenne and Becker muscular dystrophies (dilated cardiomyopathy), Emery–Dreifuss muscular dystrophy and myotonic dystrophy (atrioventricular conduction defects). Oculopharyngeal muscular dystrophy typically presents in later life with slowly progressive ptosis and dysphagia. It is not associated with cardiac involvement.

201

Muscle disease is a feature of hypothyroidism, hyperthyroidism, hypokalaemia and Cushing's syndrome (including secondary to corticosteroid therapy). Isolated hyperglycaemia is not associated with a myopathy.

Quick fix: Causes of drug-induced myopathy

- Acute/subacute myopathy:
  - cholesterol-lowering drugs
  - opiates
  - amiodarone
  - cyclosporin
  - beta-blockers
- Acute rhabdomyolysis:
  - opiates
  - cocaine
  - amphetamines

- Chronic painless myopathy:
  - corticosteroids
  - chloroquine
  - amiodarone
  - colchicine
- Inflammatory myopathy:
  - D-penicillamine
  - procainamide
- Hypokalaemic myopathy:
  - diuretics
  - purgatives

Sleep disorders

202 All of the following are recognised clinical features of narcolepsy *except*:

a disrupted night-time sleep

b cataplexy

c hypnagogic hallucinations

d sleep paralysis

e autonomic neuropathy.

203 Which of the following statements about narcolepsy is *incorrect*?

a 90% of Caucasian patients with confirmed narcolepsy and cataplexy are HLA DQ B1 *0602 positive.

b It is associated with high levels of hypocretin (orexin) in the CSF in the majority of cases.

c It may present in childhood.

d Patients may resume driving after contacting the DVLA if they respond to treatment.

e Clomipramine is of use in the treatment of associated cataplexy.

204 Which of the following statements about the sleep cycle is correct?

a   Newborns spend less than 30% of total sleep time in REM sleep.

b   REM sleep periods get shorter as the night's sleep progresses.

c   There is no inhibition of muscle tone in REM sleep in healthy adults.

d   Benzodiazepines reduce the proportion of REM sleep.

e   Narcolepsy patients rarely enter REM sleep within 15 minutes of sleep onset.

205 Which of the following statements about restless legs syndrome is *incorrect*?

a   It may be associated with iron-deficiency anaemia.

b   It responds to treatment with levodopa.

c   A peripheral neuropathy can be identified in the majority of cases.

d   It can cause daytime as well as nocturnal symptoms.

e   There is a recognised association with uraemia.

202

Narcolepsy classically presents with a tetrad of symptoms, including excessive daytime sleepiness, cataplexy, hypnagogic hallucinations and sleep paralysis. Patients often complain of disturbed night-time sleep. Autonomic neuropathy is not a feature of narcolepsy.

203

Narcolepsy may present in the first decade of life, and diagnosis may be difficult. Recently, a canine model of inherited narcolepsy was linked to mutations in the receptor for a neurotransmitter, hypocretin. Neurons containing hypocretin are found in the human hypothalamus, and are frequently reduced in number in narcoleptic brains. CSF hypocretin levels are low or absent in human narcolepsy, but this is also the case in other conditions, so its use as a diagnostic test is not validated. Over 90% of Caucasian patients with narcolepsy and cataplexy have HLA DQ B1 *0602.

204

REM (rapid eye movement) sleep forms part of the normal sleep cycle, and is usually reached after passing through light phases of sleep (stages I and II) into deeper sleep (stages III and IV). Narcolepsy patients typically experience sleep-onset REM activity. Newborns spend approximately 50% of total sleep time in REM sleep, but this proportion decreases with age to approximately 25% in healthy young adults. Muscle tone is inhibited during REM sleep. Benzodiazepines reduce the proportion of time spent in REM sleep.

205

The symptoms of restless legs syndrome (RLS) are characteristically nocturnal. Discomfort in the legs leads to an irresistible urge to move the legs, which may temporarily relieve the discomfort. RLS may be associated with iron-deficiency anaemia, uraemia and pregnancy. A small proportion of cases are associated with peripheral neuropathy.

Quick fix: The Epworth Sleepiness Scale

Give a score of 0 to 3 (where 1 = slight chance, 2 = moderate chance and 3 = high chance) for the likelihood that you would fall asleep in each of the situations listed below.

1 Sitting and reading
2 Watching television
3 Sitting inactive in a public place
4 As a passenger in a car for an hour without a break
5 Lying down to rest in the afternoon
6 Sitting and talking to someone
7 Sitting quietly after lunch (no alcohol)
8 In a car, stopped in traffic

Normal range (6–10)
Narcolepsy range (13–24)

Quick fix: Causes of excessive daytime sleepiness

- Sleep deprivation
- Obstructive sleep apnoea
- Central sleep apnoea
- Narcolepsy
- Idiopathic CNS hypersomnia
- Other CNS disorders (e.g. encephalitis, stroke, tumour)
- Psychiatric disorders
- Drugs (e.g. anti-epileptic medication)

Neurogenetics

206 The following are genetic disorders with prominent neurological involvement. Which one occurs much less commonly in females than in males?

a Wilson's disease

b von Recklinghausen's disease (neurofibromatosis type I)

c Friedreich's ataxia

d Duchenne's muscular dystrophy

e Huntington's disease.

207 All of the following diseases are associated with a pathological trinucleotide repeat expansion *except*:

a Friedreich's ataxia

b Huntington's disease

c fragile X mental retardation

d myotonic dystrophy

e familial Alzheimer's disease.

208 With regard to transmission of the mitochondrial MELAS 3243 mutation, which of the following statements is true?

a Male-to-male transmission is common.

b Phenotypic manifestation of the disease is affected by heteroplasmy.

c Spontaneous mutations account for > 90% of cases.

d The mutation is in a nuclear gene encoding a subunit of complex I.

e One copy of the gene is present in each mitochondrion.

209 A 25-year-old man consults you because he is worried about the risk of transmitting Huntington's disease to his 3-year-old daughter. His maternal uncle has recently been diagnosed with Huntington's disease at the age of 67 years. His mother is currently 50 years old and has no symptoms. His maternal grandmother died in a psychiatric hospital after developing dementia and chorea. Which of the following statements is true?

a The daughter should be tested for the repeat expansion immediately to ascertain her risk of developing the disease.

b If the patient tests positive for the gene mutation, it will be necessary to test his mother to confirm the diagnosis.

c Without knowing any further test results, the risk to his child of carrying the Huntington's gene is approximately 12%.

d The risk to the daughter is negligible, because male-to-female transmission cannot occur in Huntington's disease.

e A normal MRI brain scan in the asymptomatic 25-year-old father would exclude him from being a carrier of the Huntington's disease gene.

206

Duchenne muscular dystrophy is an
X-linked recessive disorder. Female
carriers of an X-linked recessive trait
may manifest the disease phenotype
under unusual circumstances, but
this is comparatively uncommon,
whereas all male carriers manifest a
pathological phenotype. The other
diseases are either autosomal
recessive (Wilson's disease,
Friedreich's ataxia) or dominant
(Huntington's disease,
neurofibromatosis type I), and so are
approximately equally common in
men and women.

207

A number of inherited neurological
diseases are associated with
trinucleotide repeat expansions. For
example, in the Huntington's disease
gene, normal alleles contain the
trinucleotide sequence C-A-G
repeated up to 35 times. Expansion
of this trinucleotide repeat such that
it is repeated more than 40 times is
sufficient to cause Huntington's
disease. Familial Alzheimer's disease
is associated with a variety of
mutations in various genes, but
none of these is an expanded
trinucleotide repeat.

208

The mitochondrion contains its own
16-kb genome that is maternally
transmitted and encodes some
subunits of the respiratory chain, and
a series of tRNAs. Each
mitochondrion contains multiple
copies of the genome, and there are
multiple mitochondria within each
cell, so the proportion of genomes
containing mutations can vary
widely between cells and tissues
(heteroplasmy). This affects whether
a disease phenotype is manifested.

209

Huntington's disease is autosomal
dominant. Although the girl's carrier
status could be easily ascertained by
gene testing, this would be entirely
unacceptable until she is old enough
to be counselled and to make an
informed decision. Her risk on the
basis of present evidence is 1:8
(12.5%). If her grandmother was
shown to carry the gene, her risk
would be 1:4, and if her father
carries the gene, her risk would be
1:2. If the father carries the gene,
then his mother is an obligate carrier.
A normal MRI brain scan does not
exclude carrier status.

Quick fix: Neurogenetic disorders associated with tri-nucleotide repeat expansions

Dominant neurological diseases (repeat encodes a polyglutamine tract in relevant protein, cell death is caused by toxic gain of function)

- Huntington's disease, dentato-rubro-pallido-luysian atrophy (DRPLA)
- Spinocerebellar ataxias (types 1, 2, 3, 6 and 7)
- X-linked bulbar and spinal muscular atrophy (Kennedy's disease)
- Oculopharyngeal muscular dystrophy

Recessive neurological diseases (repeat in non-coding sequence abolishes expression of relevant protein)

- Friedreich's ataxia
- Fragile X syndrome (X-linked learning disability)

Dominant multisystem disease (repeat in non-coding sequence, mechanism of disease uncertain)

- Myotonic dystrophy

Quick fix: Diseases associated with mitochondrial DNA mutations

Disease	Inheritance	Clinical features	RRF in muscle	Type of mutation
LHON	Maternal transmission	Subacute bilateral optic neuropathy; male predominance (4:1)	No	Point mutation
MELAS	Maternal transmission	Short stature; migraine-like headache; stroke-like episodes; hearing loss; partial and generalised seizures; basal ganglia calcification	Yes	Point mutation
MERRF	Maternal transmission	Myoclonus; generalised seizures; ataxia; deafness; myopathy; dementia; optic atrophy	Yes	Point mutation
CPEO	Sporadic (occasionally maternal)	External ophthalmoplegia and ptosis; occasionally proximal myopathy	Yes	Deletion
KSS	Sporadic	CPEO; retinitis pigmentosa; onset before age 20 years; ataxia; heart block, CSF protein >1 g/L; myopathy; dementia; diabetes mellitus	Yes	Deletion

LHON, Leber's hereditary optic neuropathy; MELAS, mitochondrial encephalopathy, lactic acidosis and stroke-like episodes; MERRF, myoclonic epilepsy with ragged red fibres; CPEO, chronic progressive external ophthalmoplegia; KSS, Kearns–Sayre syndrome; RRF, ragged red fibres.

Developmental disorders of the nervous system

210 Which of the following is *not* characteristically seen in type I Arnold–Chiari malformation?

a   downbeat nystagmus

b   dizziness provoked by head movement

c   cough headache

d   syringomyelia

e   myelomeningocoele.

211 Which of the following definitions of cortical malformations is *incorrect*?

a   Lissencephaly – multiple enlarged sulci.

b   Heterotopia – a misplaced collection of neurons and glia.

c   Polymicrogyria – multiple thin small gyri.

d   Schizencephaly – infolding of cortical grey matter along a hemispheric cleft.

e   Cortical dysplasia – thickened cortex with loss of the grey–white matter junction.

212 Which of the following is *not* a well-recognised maternal risk factor for the development of a fetus with a neural-tube defect?

a anti-epileptic drugs

b cigarette smoking

c previous pregnancy complicated by neural-tube defect

d folate deficiency

e diabetes mellitus.

213 Which of the following is *not* a recognised component of Sturge–Weber syndrome?

a port-wine naevus in the territory of the ophthalmic division of the trigeminal nerve

b hemiparesis

c tramline calcification seen on plain skull radiograph

d hemihypertrophy

e epilepsy.

210

Type I Arnold–Chiari malformation is associated with a relative normal fourth ventricle and a low incidence of associated myelomeningocoele. Sagittal MRI imaging shows extension of the cerebellar tonsils below the foramen magnum. Some cases have an associated cervical syrinx.

211

Disorders of cortical development are an important cause of epilepsy. Several single-gene disorders underlying these conditions have been identified, and pathogenic mutations have been demonstrated in the genes encoding *doublecortin, reelin* and *filamin-1*. Lissencephaly refers to the macroscopic appearance of smooth brain, caused by absent gyri and sulci.

212

Couples who have one child with a neural-tube defect have a 1 in 40 chance of having another baby with the same defect. This risk rises to 1 in 20 if two previous children have been affected by the condition. Neural-tube defects are also associated with folate deficiency, anti-epileptic drugs (particularly sodium valproate) and maternal diabetes. There is no association between maternal smoking and neural-tube defects.

213

Sturge–Weber syndrome refers to the association of a vascular naevus in the distribution of the ophthalmic division of the trigeminal nerve with cerebral calcification that is best seen on plain skull films and CT scans performed after the second year of life. Patients frequently develop partial seizures on the side opposite to the naevus, with increasing hemiparesis and impaired growth of the arm and leg.

Quick fix: Classification and clinical features of Arnold–Chiari malformation

	Chiari type I	*Chiari type II*
Neuroanatomy	Bilateral herniation of cerebellar tonsils through foramen magnum	Inferior displacement of medulla, fourth ventricle and cerebellar vermis through foramen magnum
Associated anomalies	Syringomyelia; hydrocephalus; platybasia	Myelomeningocoele and hydrocephalus (invariable); cortical malformation
Age at presentation	Variable – often presents in adult life (third and fourth decades)	Infancy
Clinical features	Cough headache; downbeat nystagmus; occasional lower cranial nerve palsies	Learning disability; progressive hydrocephalus requiring shunting; lower cranial nerve palsies

Neurological complications of systemic disease

214 Which of the following statements about neurological complications of glucose metabolism is *incorrect*?

a Insulinoma may present initially with a generalised tonic–clonic convulsion.

b Hyperglycaemia may present with focal motor seizures.

c Hypoglycaemic attacks may cause focal neurological deficits.

d The hippocampus is relatively protected from the effects of severe hypoglycaemia.

e Cerebral oedema is a recognised complication of the treatment of diabetic ketoacidosis.

215 Which of the following is *not* a recognised association between systemic disease and cranial nerve palsy?

a primary hypothyroidism and abducens (VI) nerve palsy

b Sjögren's syndrome and sensory trigeminal (V) neuropathy

c diabetes mellitus and oculomotor (III) nerve palsy

d sarcoidosis and optic (II) neuropathy

e Lyme disease and facial (VII) nerve palsy.

216 Which of the following statements about pregnancy and neurological disorders is correct?

a   The risk of fetal abnormalities in patients taking anti-epileptic drugs is 1–2%.

b   Pregnancy is characteristically associated with an improvement in idiopathic intracranial hypertension.

c   Spinal meningiomata commonly regress during pregnancy.

d   Symptoms from carpal tunnel syndrome frequently improve during pregnancy.

e   Cerebral venous sinus thrombosis is commonest during the third trimester and in the postpartum period.

217 Which of the following is not a recognised complication of chronic alcohol dependence?

a   chronic inflammatory demyelinating polyneuropathy

b   Wernicke's encephalopathy

c   cerebellar ataxia

d   acute necrotising myopathy

e   central pontine myelinolysis.

214

Metabolic disturbances secondary to diabetes mellitus present with a variety of neurological abnormalities, including coma, delirium, focal motor seizures and generalised convulsions. The hippocampus is particularly vulnerable to damage as a result of severe hypoglycaemia.

215

Hypothyroidism may be associated with hearing loss but is not associated with extraocular muscle palsy. In contrast, Graves' disease may present with exophthalmos and an ocular myopathy particularly affecting the medial and inferior recti, causing restriction in abduction and up-gaze.

216

Pregnancy is likely to exacerbate the symptoms of carpal tunnel syndrome. Idiopathic intracranial hypertension may present during pregnancy, typically during the first trimester. The risk of fetal malformations in patients taking anti-epileptic drugs is approximately 8–10%. Spinal meningiomata may expand rapidly during pregnancy, and this is believed to be due to tumour-cell expression of oestrogen receptors.

217

Alcohol is associated with a wide range of neurological complications. The polyneuropathy is characteristically axonal rather than demyelinating.

Quick fix: Alcohol and the nervous system

Acute intoxication

Withdrawal

- Seizures
- Delirium tremens
- Hallucinosis

Chronic alcohol intoxication/nutritional deficiency

- Forebrain:
  - Wernicke's encephalopathy
  - Korsakoff's (amnestic) syndrome
  - Marchiafava–Bignami syndrome (destruction of myelin in corpus callosum and anterior commissure)
  - cerebral atrophy
  - dementia
  - optic neuropathy
  - increased susceptibility to subdural haematoma and ischaemic stroke
  - hepatic encephalopathy

- Hindbrain:
  - cerebellar degeneration (Purkinje cell loss in anterior and superior vermis)
  - central pontine myelinolysis
- Neuromuscular:
  - motor and sensory axonal peripheral neuropathy
  - pellagra
  - acute necrotising myopathy
  - chronic myopathy

Fact finder

Note: Two references systems are used. Numbers in ordinary type are page numbers with a single page number pointing to 'quick fix' information. Numbers in **bold** type are question numbers. 'vs' indicates the differentiation of two conditions.

Fact finder

Fact finder

Fact finder

Fact finder

Fact finder

Fact finder